BARNES & NOBLE HEALTH BASICS™

Migraine

By Joan Raymond

D1166300

BARNES
&NOBLE
BOOKS
NEW YORK

About the Author

Joan Raymond is the author, editor, or contributing writer of numerous articles on health, fitness, and medicine.

About the Contributors

Portions of this work were reviewed by Stephen Possick, M.D. and David Weisman, M.D. The nutritional information was written by Mindy Hermann, R.D. The information about complementary therapies was written by Melanie Hulse. The information on meditation and biofeedback was written by Lawrence Edwards, Ph.D.

Barbara J. Morgan Publisher
Barnes & Noble Basics

Barb Chintz Editorial Director
Barbara Rietschel Art Director
Clellen Bryant Editor
Emily Seese Editorial Assistant
Della R. Mancuso Production Manager

Illustrations by Cynthia Saniewski

Table of Contents

Foreword

If you or a loved one has just received a diagnosis of migraine, the first thing you will want to know is how to manage the condition effectively. This is where Barnes & Noble Health Basics *Migraine* comes in. Written with expert guidance from leading physicians, this informative book leads you to a deeper understanding of your symptoms and treatment.

No matter what type of migraine you get, you'll find plenty of useful information on treatment, medication, nutrition, complementary therapies, searching the Internet, and putting together a health care team. You'll also get the latest news on cutting-edge research and some wise advice on the role of stress and comfort in managing your health.

With all of these helpful insights at your fingertips, you'll be able to take control of your migraine and become an advocate for your own health care. Remember: An informed patient is an empowered one. So read on to put yourself in the driver's seat when it comes to treating and managing your migraine.

Barb Chintz
Editorial Director
Barnes & Noble Health Basics Series

CHAPTER 1

Getting the Diagnosis

Experiencing the symptoms
signals as subtle as a marching band in your head

What does it feel like to have a migraine? It can start out innocently enough. Perhaps you take a bite of some chocolate or have an after-work glass of wine. Most of the time, that doesn't create a problem. But then maybe once a month, or once a week, seemingly out of nowhere, your senses go into overdrive. Your head pounds; the slightest noise is agony; you shield your eyes to block out any light. You may feel nauseated, nervous, exhausted—a whole gamut of symptoms. Obviously, this is not a simple headache. This is the kind of misery that makes you want to draw the blinds and collapse in a fetal position in a corner. If it's any comfort, you are not alone. In the United States, approximately 18 percent of women get migraines, and 6 percent of men get migraines.

After a few hours or perhaps a day, the dreadful all-encompassing pain passes and you return to your old self, a bit dazed, but functioning. You get back to your old routine—that is until the head pain strikes again. What is going on? If the pattern continues, chances are you go to your doctor and complain of head pain, perhaps nausea. Most likely your doctor will start to question you about the specifics of your plight. When did this first start? Where is the pain? How long does it last? The answers to these questions are vital. The problem is that most people don't pay the right kind of attention to their bodies, so they don't know how to talk effectively to their doctors about their symptoms. Doctors have to read between the lines. Not surprisingly, whenever a doctor and a patient talk, there can be miscommunication. Think back to the time your car was on the fritz. Remember how you tried to explain the clunk-clunk noise to your mechanic and how he looked at you quizzically? Well, sometimes, talking to your doctor about your headache symptoms is just as difficult. Even those who are in tune with their bodies are amazed at how hard it is to be specific about various types of pain.

What can you do about this communication gap? For starters, you need to know what symptoms can arise with the disease known as **migraine**. Having several of these symptoms does not mean that you have a migraine, but it does mean that you need to talk to your doctor about them.

Common Symptoms of Migraine

Pain: Moderate to severe pulsating head pain (generally, but not always, restricted to one side of the head, directly behind the eyes, or around the eyes). This pain usually increases with body movement.

Sensory symptoms: Sensitivity to light, sounds, and smells. Visual problems, such as seeing flashing lights, or partially blocked vision. Blurred vision.

Body symptoms: Nausea, no appetite, fatigue, feeling intensely hot or cold, excessive sweating. Scalp tightness or tenderness.

Psychological symptoms: Abrupt changes in mood, feeling especially nervous or irritable. Problems concentrating. Language confusion. Also feeling drowsy or hyperaware.

Red Flags for Headache

If you experience any of these symptoms, call your doctor immediately or go to the emergency room.

- ◆ Headache with a fever.
- ◆ Headache when you bend your chin to your chest.
- ◆ Headache with blurred vision, slurred speech, and/or numbness in the arms or legs.
- ◆ Sudden onset of "new" severe headache.

Seeing your doctor
be your own best advocate

To begin, your doctor will take your medical history. This will help determine whether a situation or illness in your past may be responsible for your pain today. (If you've had any type of head scans, for any reason, let him know.) More general questions will explore your overall health, lifestyle, emotional status, and family history of headache.

If your doctor suspects migraine, then one of the first things he will do is ask you a slew of diagnostic questions. Help your doctor by providing as much detail as possible about the attack, including when the pain began and when it stopped, and if there was specific activity you were doing at the time of the attack. Tell him if you were nauseated. If you took any over-the-counter medicine for the pain. Whether you had to miss work because of the intensity of the attack. Don't spare any detail. When it comes to your health, there is no such thing as trivial information.

Just Three Questions

◆ Has a headache limited your activities for a day or more in the last three months?

◆ Are you nauseated or sick to your stomach when you have a headache?

◆ Does light bother you when you have a headache?

According to the American Headache Society, two "yes" answers to these three questions suggests a high likelihood of migraine. An analysis determined that of patients who answered "yes" to two of the three questions, 93 percent were determined by headache experts to be suffering from migraine. Though the questions will obviously not identify all people with migraine, they do provide a simple guide for patients and physicians attempting to diagnose migraine.

Sample Questions

◆ How long and how often have you been having headaches?

◆ How old were you when you first had this type of headache?

◆ Where is the pain? The site or sites of pain—one side, both sides?

◆ How long does it last? You need to establish the time from onset (that first twinge) to peak pain to cessation of pain.

◆ Can you describe the pain? Is it throbbing or pulsing? Is the pain mild, moderate, or severe and disabling?

◆ Does minor movement increase the pain?

◆ How does the headache begin? Do you have any advance warning, such as nausea, vomiting, sensitivity to light and noise, weakness on one side of the body, visual blind spots or zigzag lines?

◆ Do light, loud noises, or strong odors make you uncomfortable or aggravate the pain?

◆ Does the headache occur at any particular time of the month? For women, menses is often a trigger for headaches. If you have been pregnant, did the headaches continue during pregnancy?

◆ Do you have a family history of headaches?

◆ Do wine, beer, chocolate, cheese, or any other foods precipitate the headache?

◆ Are you taking any prescription or over-the-counter medication?

◆ Have you had a head injury?

◆ Have you been having any eye problems, such as a change in your vision?

◆ Do you have any other medical conditions?

Similarities to other disorders
ruling out other possibilities

As your doctor listens to your symptoms, he will be lining up all the possible disorders and diseases that match your symptoms. He will then start eliminating them one by one, until he settles on the disorder or disease that explains your symptoms.

Migraine symptoms can mimic everything from premenstrual syndrome to stroke. (For the record, fewer than one percent of headaches are due to a brain tumor or stroke.) The key to successful treatment is a proper evaluation of your headache pain. You may think that all headache pain is the same. It isn't. Your doctor will ask you some very specific questions and see if your symptoms fit with any of the following health problems:

Tension headaches
This head pain is most likely due to tension in the neck and scalp muscles. The pain is bilateral, meaning both sides of the head are affected. These muscles often contract during intense activity or stressful situations, producing non-throbbing pressure-like pain. There is no change in ability to function. Tension headaches usually get better after a few hours.

Cluster headaches
These are severe headaches that last on average about 45 minutes and typically affect one side of the head. These headaches come in clusters, meaning they come in bouts, anywhere from several times a day to several times a week or month.

Analgesic rebound headaches
This type of head pain comes from taking many daily doses of analgesics, especially short-acting ones. (For more on this, see page 58.)

Sinus headaches

A sinus infection can cause intense throbbing pain under the eyes and along the eyebrows. The pain worsens when bending over. These headaches are usually associated with other symptoms of sinusitis, such as fever and discolored nasal discharge.

When doctors can't quite pin down the head pain, they may explore the role of stress in your life. (If you are a woman, they may consider your head pain as part and parcel of your menstrual cycle.)

Headache and stress: When your body reacts to acute stress, you usually experience some very distinct bodily changes: Your heart races to increase blood to the muscles; your breathing increases to get more oxygen to the brain so it stays alert; and your digestion shuts down in order to send energy to the muscles. These are just a few of the responses that are hard-wired into your body to help it handle a stressful situation. Once the stress has passed, your body then returns to its normal restful state. But what happens if you have repeated exposure to stressful situations? Researchers think that chronic stress, the curse of the modern age, can trigger or worsen a number of health problems, such as migraines. The problem is that the symptoms of stress often mimic the symptoms of migraine so it's easy to put the blame on stress, instead of on the underlying migraine disease that chronic stress may have kickstarted. For more on stress, see Chapter 11.

Headaches and the menstrual cycle: Headaches are often associated with premenstrual syndrome or PMS. This syndrome includes nausea, headache, and loss of appetite. The situation is further complicated by the fact that migraines in some women are triggered by their period. Hence the name: menstrual migraines. See Chapter 4 for more information.

Getting the diagnosis
it's trickier than you think

For all the agony that migraines inflict, thousands of individuals do not get the proper diagnosis and therefore are unable to get proper treatment. To be fair, migraine diagnosis is not as straightforward as you might think. There's no specific blood test, no ultrasound or X-ray to determine whether you have the disease, though sometimes doctors do order imaging tests of the brain, such as a CT scan or MRI. This does not mean you have a brain tumor!

The diagnosis for migraine is made by carefully assessing your symptoms, performing an evaluation, and getting your medical history. Then all this information is weighed against the criteria for migraine as well as for other disorders that cause headaches. If this isn't done, it's possible to have your migraine pain dismissed as a tension headache, sinusitis, or stress. This misdiagnosis compounds an already miserable situation because you don't get medication for your pain. Or, if you do, the medication prescribed is not appropriate for the treatment of migraine pain. The American Medical Association analyzed survey data from more than 20,000 individuals, 12 to 80 years of age. Of those who met the diagnostic criteria for migraine, only 41 percent of women and 29 percent of men reported having received a medical diagnosis of migraine.

Auras

Auras are symptoms that usually occur 30 to 60 minutes before a migraine headache begins. Auras develop gradually over 5 to 20 minutes and usually last less than one hour. Sometimes auras fade as the headache pain begins, or they may persist in the early stages. Common aura symptoms are visual disturbances, areas of lost or reduced vision; zigzag lines, sparks, stars, and flashes before the eyes; distortions of objects; haziness or shimmering of objects; blindness in half of the visual field of one eye. Some people attribute Picasso's paintings of fractured faces, with noses and eyes crazily shifted from their usual places, to the fact that he got migraines.

The International Headache Society has established the standards for migraine diagnosis. The following lists are dervived from their work.

Criteria for Common Migraine

◆ At least two or more headache attacks that last 4 to 72 hours (untreated or unsuccessfully treated).

◆ Headache has at least two of the following characteristics: Unilateral site (one side of the head). Pulsating quality. Moderate to severe intensity. Aggravation caused by walking, climbing stairs, or similar physical activity.

◆ During headache, at least one of these symptoms occurs: Nausea or vomiting (or both), photophobia (sensitivity to light), and phono-phobia (sensitivity to sound). No evidence of related organic disease.

Criteria for Migraine with Aura or "Classic Migraine"

◆ At least two attacks with at least three of these four characteristics:

◆ One or more fully reversible aura symptoms occur, indicating brain dysfunction. (Don't be scared."Brain dysfunction"is a medical term that simply means your brain processing is temporarily compromised. The visual disturbance of the aura is a type of brain dysfunction. The "dysfunction" is not permanent, and your mental or physical capacity is not permanently damaged.)

◆ At least one aura symptom develops gradually over a time period of more than 4 minutes, or two or more symptoms occur in succession. No single aura symptom lasts more than 60 minutes.

◆ Headache follows aura with a free interval of less than 60 minutes (it may also begin before or simultaneously with the aura). No evidence of related organic disease.

Keeping a headache journal
the first step in understanding your migraine

One of the best ways to keep tabs on your symptoms is to record them in a health journal. By noting your daily symptoms for several weeks, you will be creating an invaluable tool that will help both you and your doctor recognize patterns that point to the right disorder. And once your disease is correctly diagnosed, keeping a health journal will be very helpful to your recovery. How so? Treatment for your migraines doesn't happen overnight. It takes time to determine the right course of treatment to ease your symptoms. By noting your symptoms, you will not only learn to pay better attention to your body and to understand what it is trying to tell you, but also to help plot the success of various treatments. Patterns will emerge, leading to the very best treatment, individualized to your particular needs. If nothing else, a journal can help you identify foods or activities that may be triggering your migraine.

Note: In the beginning, it's a good idea to keep track of your health on a daily basis for several weeks. The reason is that many people who get migraines experience some unusual symptoms a day or so before the agonizing pain of the headache sets in.

Set up your sheet of paper—or notebook or journal—following these guidelines.

Date: Simply date the page, and write down how you're feeling. If it's a good day, great! Tell your diary. But if you're feeling a little achy or just plain out of sorts, write that down, too.

Duration of pain: How long did the headache last?

Location: Is the pain on one side of the head or on both sides? Does it move?

Pain: Dull, throbbing, pulsing, knifelike? Rate the pain on a scale of 0 to 3, with 0 being pain-free, 1 mild, 2 moderate, and 3 severe.

Emotions: What were you feeling before the onset of the headache? Were you angry or stressed? As you know, migraines are not an emotional illness. But emotions and stress can play a part in how you are feeling and can impact your head pain.

Activities: What were you doing right before the attack? Exercising? Sleeping? Working?

Food: What did you eat in the 24 hours prior to your headache? You may uncover food triggers that set off your headache.

Medication: Write down all over-the-counter and prescription medications you take for the pain, including dosage and frequency. Include the time you took the medicine, whether it worked, and when and if there were any side effects.

Quality of life: Did you have to miss work during a headache episode? Are you missing out on social activities? Let your doctor know. Quality of life is an important part of overall good health.

For women: What day does the headache fall in your menstrual cycle? How many days since your last period?

What is a migraine?
understanding this chronic disorder

Yes, migraine is a chronic illness, but in reality it is an illness that strikes episodically. That differentiates it from a chronic illness like diabetes where you must deal with the illness every day by checking your blood sugar levels. Migraine is also one of the earliest recorded medical conditions known to man. The first thing to understand is that migraine is not an illness caused by an inability to cope with the common stresses of life. You are not weak. And you are in no way to blame for developing this condition.

Although doctors have not yet determined the exact cause of the disease, they have linked the migraine to specific changes in the brain. During a migraine attack, blood vessels in and around the brain can become inflamed, and the neurochemistry of pain perception is changed. In the past, pain was considered the result of some kind of physical action—an injury, an inflammation, an infection, a fever. But new research suggests pain is not just a *physical* response, but a complex phenomenon that involves the whole person—body and mind. Thus, pain affects your emotions, your ability to focus your attention, and your memory. This new pain theory helps to explain why a sudden flash of anger or an unpleasant memory can set off a migraine.

Migraine Triggers

How do migraines happen? Many people with migraines say that their headaches are set off by certain **triggers**. Some migraine triggers, such as diet, are controllable to a certain degree. Others, such as changing weather patterns, aren't controllable. Sometimes triggers instigate a migraine immediately; in other cases, the migraine doesn't come on for a few hours. There are no hard and fast rules about triggers; they vary from one person to the another. Moreover, every migraine can be different. The three basic categories of triggers are dietary, environmental, and physiological.

Dietary Triggers Food, beverage, and preservative triggers include aged cheese, alcohol (especially red wine), aspartame (an artificial sweetener), citrus fruits, chocolate, coconut and coconut oil (even the smell of suntan lotion can trigger a migraine in some people), coffee, dairy products, food preservatives such as MSG, nitrates (often used as preservatives in luncheon meats), nuts, olive oil, salt, sulfites (used as preservatives in a long list of foods from baked goods to pickles to trail mix).

Enviromental Triggers These include loud, repetitive noises, glare, strong odors (such as too much perfume), changing weather patterns or specific weather conditions such as dry winds, altitude changes, air pollution, second-hand smoke, even the flicker of a computer monitor.

Physiological Triggers These can include too much or too little sleep, skipped meals, hypoglycemia (low blood sugar), menstruation, fatigue, physical activity, and stress.

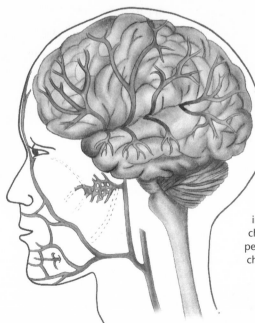

The brain is surrounded by numerous blood vessels. During a migraine attack, blood vessels in and around the brain can become inflamed, and the neuro-chemistry of pain perception is changed.

me, why now?
there are some reasons

Everyone reacts differently to a diagnosis of a chronic disorder like migraine. For those who have been plagued with uncomfortable symptoms for a long time, there may be relief and then a whole host of feelings, from fear and anger to sadness and resignation. The good news is that migraine can be treated and controlled. In fact, the best thing to do is to view this health news as just another of life's challenges that you can manage. You are not good or bad for getting this disorder. You did nothing to cause it. It simply happens. Your task now is to learn how to partner with your doctor to manage your new disorder and live your life to the fullest. More on this on pages 95-108.

Know that you are not alone. According to the National Headache Foundation (NHF), migraine is more common than asthma, diabetes or even congestive heart failure. And chances are pretty good that if you have migraines, a family member probably has migraines too. According to the NHF, migraines seem to run in families. About 70 percent of those who get migraines have a hereditary influence. If one parent has a history of migraines, a child has about a 50 percent chance of developing migraines at some point. But if both mom and dad have migraines, the chance of a child developing migraines at some point jumps to a whopping 75 percent.

A great many famous people, past and present, have had migraines. Back in the days of the Roman Empire, Caesar had migraines; so did the apostle Paul. The philosopher Immanuel Kant had migraines, as did Freud, the father of psychotherapy. Author Lewis Carroll experienced migraines, as did Elvis Presley.

Some current famous people who know all about migraine are the TV show *Friends'* star Lisa Kudrow, football great Terrell Davis, and basketball legend Kareem Abdul Jabaar. And if you want to know how you can laugh at the disease, follow Whoopi Goldberg's lead. The renowned writer Joan Didion, in fact, wrote a very moving essay called "In Bed" describing her migraines. If these creative and productive people can manage with migraines, you can too.

FIRST PERSON INSIGHTS

Getting over the fear

"The first time I had a migraine I wanted to die. I was nauseated, the light was killing my eyes, and I couldn't even listen to the radio. I was only 25 years old, and I thought I had a brain tumor. But I did nothing since the pain went away after a day. I figured I just had a really, really bad headache. I didn't have another attack for several months. That pain lasted for several days, and I really started to get scared. But I still didn't tell my doctor about the headaches—even when I would go in for routine physicals. I was afraid they were due to something awful, and I didn't want to know about it.

After one particularly bad attack when my vision went completely haywire, I finally screwed up my courage and called my doctor for a special appointment. That was five years after my very first attack. My doctor was amazed at my silence. After listening to my symptoms, he assured me that I didn't have a brain tumor. In fact, he said my dad used to get the same kind of headaches. I hadn't remembered that. I've been getting migraine treatment for the last three years, and I feel great. I still get migraines, but not so frequently, maybe one or two a year. Seeing my doctor put me back in control. That's the greatest feeling in the world."

—Ellen S., Cleveland, OH

You are not alone
the big picture of migraine

Migraines occur across the spectrum of race, personality types and social groups. Here are some fascinating statistics about the disease compiled from the American Migraine Study II, a population-based survey conducted in 1999 for the National Headache Foundation. The comprehensive findings of American Migraine Study II—A Ten Year Report Card, were published in Headache in 2001.

◆ Migraines affect about 13 percent of the population aged 12 and older.

◆ About 80 percent of those with migraine rate their headaches as severe or extremely severe.

◆ More than 20 percent have sought treatment for migraines in an emergency room.

◆ More than 50 percent of those with migraine say that when they experience an episode, they also experience a 50 percent or greater reduction in productivity, both in work and/or school.

◆ Almost 40 percent of those with migraine say the pain is so severe they must take to their beds.

◆ Only about half of respondents (who met the clinical definition of migraine) report ever having had their condition diagnosed by a doctor.

◆ About 60 percent of those with migraine say they still use only over-the-counter medications for treatment.

◆ More than 40 percent of migraine sufferers report headache pain five or more days in the last three months.

Researchers know that migraines are most commonly found in women, with about a three-to-one female-to-male ratio. In children, however, migraines are much more common in boys than in girls. Migraine also seems to have a life span. Though the first episode may be in childhood, the incidence of migraine increases during adolescence. About 80 percent of those who develop migraines will have their first episode by age 30, and their migraines will generally continue through their 30s and 40s. Though a migraine can begin at any age, they are less likely to start after the age of 50. And with increased age, episodes of migraine may decrease in severity and frequency.

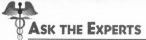

ASK THE EXPERTS

Is my brain normal?

Of course it is. Though a great deal happens to the brain during a migraine, the changes in brain function are not permanent. It is, however, very important to get your migraine assessed and then treated. Some research suggests that frequent, untreated migraine episodes may change the pain centers in the brain, leading to chronic head pain.

Is there any cure for migraines?

So far medication can only provide symptom relief, interrupt a migraine in process, and/or reduce the frequency of migraines. Many people with migraine find relief in over-the-counter or prescription medication and in complementary therapies such as acupuncture or biofeedback.

Do I have a migraine personality?

This is one of the most common myths about migraine. People who get migraines can be uptight or relaxed. They can be perfectionists or slobs, shy or the life of the party. That said, there is an association between migraine and anxiety, depression, and panic attacks.

Migraine 911
what you can do right now for relief

The pain of a migraine is unbearable: "It's like a poker in my eye;" "I feel as if a train is going through my head;" "If I move a fraction of an inch, I will throw up." While there are a number of medications and therapies for you and your doctor to consider (see pages 45-66, 141-162), there are certain simple things you can do right now that will help you get through the day:

- ◆ Apply cold compresses or ice packs to your head.

- ◆ Conversely, try a warm wet towel on your head.

- ◆ Drink a cup of coffee or a can of caffeinated soda.

- ◆ Take a hot shower.

- ◆ If the pain is in one eye, wear an eye patch over that eye.

- ◆ Have migraine medication on hand.

- ◆ Arrange in advance for backup if you need help taking care of small children, elderly parents, or pets.

- ◆ Create a migraine safety zone in your house or apartment that is noise and light free.

- ◆ Apply pressure to acupressure wrist points. See page 154 for instructions.

- ◆ Practice deep breathing. See page 143 for instructions.

- ◆ Avoid eating until pain has passed.

- ◆ Drink plenty of water.

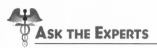

I always grab a can of soda when I feel a migraine coming on. Why is that?

At the first sign of a headache, many people unconsciously drink a cup of tea, coffee, or a can of soda. The key ingredient they are seeking is caffeine. This natural drug, found in coffee, teas, and chocolate, can cause blood vessels to constrict. It also speeds the action of analgesics, such as aspirin and acetaminophen. This is why many over-the-counter remedies for headaches include caffeine in their ingredients.

FIRST PERSON INSIGHTS

Don't overdo the medicine

"The pain of my migraine was so bad that I confess I got really desperate. My doctor had given me a prescription for my migraines so I immediately took two pills and prayed for relief. When nothing happened after an hour, I took two more. Still nothing, so I tried some over-the-counter migraine pills. That's when things went from bad to awful. I got violently sick and couldn't stop shaking or throwing up. It was the worst experience of my life. I realized then I needed help fast. I called my doctor who had me go to the emergency room. They put me on intravenous fluid and something to help with the nausea. I felt much better in a few hours. After that, I saw a neurologist who worked out a very specific plan of treatment. He explained to me that if one pill is good, two is not better, and three is downright dangerous."

—Jay W., Somers, NY

Helpful resources

Heal Your Headache: The 1-2-3 Program for Taking Charge of Your Pain
by David Buchholz and Stephen G. Reich

No More Headaches No More Migraines
by Zuzana Bic

The Women's Migraine Survival Guide: The Most Complete, Up-To-Date Resource on the Causes of Your Migraine Pain— And Treatments for Real Relief
by Christina Peterson and Christine Adamec

Migraine
by Oliver W. Sacks

Headache Help: A Complete Guide to Understanding Headaches and the Medications That Relieve Them
Fully revised and updated by Susan Lang and Lawrence Robbins

The Chronic Illness Workbook
by Patricia Fennel

"In Bed," by Joan Didion, from her book *The White Album*

National Headache Foundation
www.headaches.org

MAGNUM
Migraine Awareness Group, a National Understanding for Migraines
www.migraines.org

American Headache Society
www.ahsnet.org

American Council for Headache Education
www.achenet.org

The International Headache Society
www.i-h-s.org

www.migraines.org
A national nonprofit group that acts as a clearinghouse for information about migraines

Migraine Explained

Unraveling the mystery
researchers are getting a clearer picture

For years, the prevailing theory about migraines was that they were caused by pressure on nerves from dilated blood vessels. Researchers dubbed this the vascular theory. But several things have happened in medicine that have forced scientists to rethink that theory. The first is tremendous improvement in brain scanning and imaging technology that has allowed doctors for the first time to see deep inside the brain and learn more about its anatomy and its function during a migraine attack. The second is the use of this technology to conduct even more sophisticated brain research focusing on the migraine.

And what scientists have concluded is that the order of events in a migraine—from the first twinge to the full-blown pain—is not as straightforward as they once believed. Today, scientists have downgraded the vascular theory from the main migraine culprit to an accomplice in the migraine process.

Though doctors still don't understand the entire sequence of events involved in the migraine, they do agree that migraine is an actual **neurovascular disorder**—meaning that your entire nervous system, including the brain and the spinal cord as well as your blood vessels—are involved in the process. That's an astounding research discovery for a disorder that's among the earliest recorded by man.

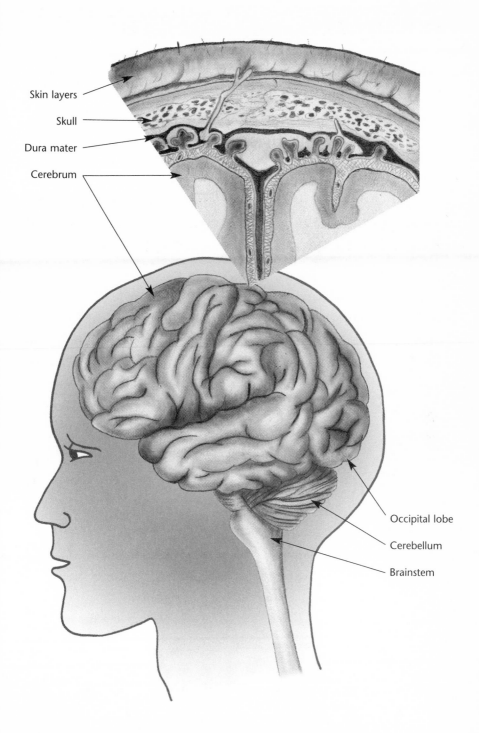

Skin layers

Skull

Dura mater

Cerebrum

Occipital lobe

Cerebellum

Brainstem

Headache vs. migraine pain
degrees of pain

You can't compare a tension headache to a severe migraine. It's like comparing a garden shovel to a bulldozer. When you have a tension headache, there are specific areas in which you experience pain, namely the scalp, with its web of highly sensitive nerves and muscles, and the muscles of the cranium. The pain you feel is mostly from muscle tension. There is no nausea, no flashing lights, and movement doesn't make it worse. An aspirin or some other over-the-counter analgesic will provide fast relief. So will a massage of the neck and the scalp.

In the case of a migraine, the process can involve the whole body, hence the nausea, sweating, vision problems, and slight numbness. The current theory of migraines is that they begin in the nerve endings, which can be found throughout the body, including the blood vessels and dura in the brain. The job of these nerve endings is to detect changes either in the environment or internally, such as temperature fluctuations, pressure changes, the presence of chemicals, and inflammation. Thus a trigger—such as changing weather patterns, a missed meal, menstruation, or a glass of wine—can set these nerve endings off. Once the nerve endings sense trouble, they signal the body's nerve cells to release special chemicals called neurotransmitters, some of which are neuropeptides. The theory is that these neurotransmitters, especially the neuropeptides, really start the ball of migraine pain rolling. Soon the entire nervous system is involved, meaning that your brain and spinal cord start to become hyper-aware to all sensations, things that most of us take for granted, like certain smells, sounds, light, or even the touch of a blanket on the skin. So much is going on during a migraine that researchers consider it a "cascade of neurological events."

The Chaos of Migraine

Most chronic illnesses have specific symptoms or physical conditions that act as their calling cards. For people with diabetes, it can be the jittery symptom of low blood sugar; for people who have hypothyroidism it is acute fatigue. For most of those who have common migraines (those are ones without the aura), there is generally no one symptom that tells them an attack is on the way. Rather, before a migraine happens, they may feel queasy, achy, or anxious or have a general feeling of disquiet—as if their whole body were in the grip of some sort of storm that is about to blow over or break wide open. The reason for the disquiet is that their whole nervous system is undergoing myriad complex changes. It is during this beginning chaotic phase that doctors advise people who have migraines to take preventive action—be it medicine, rest, whatever works—to avert a full-blown storm known in the medical world as the migraine.

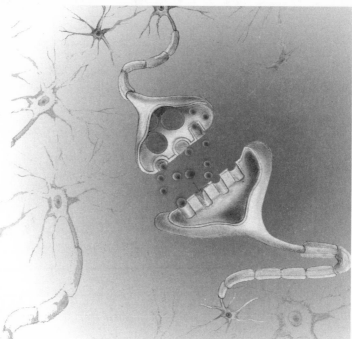

Chemical messengers, called neurotransmitters (shown here in green), are sent from one nerve fiber to another. Normally, these neurotransmitters are released from tiny notches at the end of one nerve fiber across a synaptic gap where they are received by a receptor.

The four stages of a migraine
from preheadache to postheadache

When people think "migraine" the first thing that comes to mind is the agonizing pain of the headache. But there is more to a migraine than that. A migraine is like a story, with a beginning, a middle, and an end. But that story is different for each and every person who experiences migraines. Not everyone will experience an episode in the same way, nor will an episode be experienced the same way each and every time. The typical migraine episode actually consists of several different parts, called phases. These phases bombard numerous body systems: gastrointestinal, neurological, sensory, and motor—just to name a few. Here is the most likely sequence of a migraine attack:

- The preheadache phase, called the **prodrome**, beginning hours or even days before the headache. This is the period when you are most vulnerable to developing a full-blown migraine.
- Sensory disturbances, called the **aura**, begin after the prodrome, lasting less than one hour. (The aura occurs in about 20 percent of people who get migraines. If you have a migraine with aura, that is called a classic migraine. A migraine without the aura is a common migraine.)
- The pain of the **headache** follows the aura and can last from one hour to three days in rare instances.
- Once pain stops, you enter the **postdrome** phase, during which you can feel fatigued or "hung over" for up to a day.

Knowing these phases and recognizing the symptoms gives you the best chance of avoiding the misery of the headache phase, because steps can be taken to stop a full-blown attack in some cases. Besides, knowing that feelings of irritability or depression are due to the migraine—not to some other illness or event—gives you control over your life, and your body.

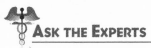

My doctor says it is really important to pay attention to the beginnings of my migraine. Why is it so important?

You need to pay attention to the prodrome stage because it is during this time that you can possibly avert a full-blown attack of migraine. This is the time to take your migraine medication. If you take it later on, it may not be effective at all.

I always seem to get a migraine right before a big event, like my son's graduation from college. How can I avoid getting migraines at these key events in my life?

Though the illness of migraine is not stress-related, stress can trigger a migraine headache. Migraines are a source of stress and stress is a source of migraines. It can be a vicious circle. Thus, the stress of anticipating a big event, such as a graduation or even a vacation, may trigger a migraine, especially if in the process you miss meals or cut back on sleep. Some people may experience migraines *after* a big event, whether a graduation or a wedding. What to do? Your doctor can work with you on finding the right treatment plan, especially since you know your triggers.

I used to get a lot of migraines when I was a teenager, but now that I have turned 45, I only get a few a year. Does that mean that my migraines are going away?

Migraines are most common between the ages 10 of and 40 but taper off after age 50. For some women, migraines may stop when you reach menopause.

The prodrome
the first stage

The prodrome (often referred to as the preheadache phase) can begin hours or even several days before a migraine headache. Think of this as the first warning sign of an impending migraine attack. About 40 percent of migraine-diagnosed patients can often prevent full-blown migraine by taking appropriate treatment during this phase.

Some of the physical symptoms include:

◆ Stiff neck

◆ A feeling of being cold (even in a warm room)

◆ Sluggishness or a sense of being tired for no apparent reason

◆ Increased thirst (Many migraine patients report feeling parched or having a "dry mouth.")

◆ Increased need to urinate

◆ Loss of appetite

◆ Fluid retention (throughout the body, but especially around the eyes)

◆ Food cravings (Though some migraine patients report loss of appetite, others can't get enough of a particular food or types of food. The cravings can be as individual as the migraine.)

◆ Light and/or sound sensitivity

The prodrome phase also includes some significant psychological and neurological symptoms that researchers are actively studying. During this phase, some migraine patients experience:

◆ Dizziness (This feeling can be very subtle, rather than an all-out attack of vertigo.)

◆ Euphoria (a sense of giddiness)

◆ Irritability

◆ Restlessness

◆ Mental sluggishness (This can also be a very subtle symptom, though some migraine patients who experience the aura have more overt problems.)

◆ Hyperactivity

◆ Fatigue and drowsiness

FIRST PERSON INSIGHTS

A 20-year misdiagnosis

"It took me a long time to get it together regarding the phases of my migraine. I've had these things for about 20 years, but I'd say it's just been in the last two years that I've come to recognize what's going on. I was misdiagnosed—everybody thought that because I'm a man I must have sinus headaches. So I wasn't even getting the right treatment. About three years ago, I tried again and went to a specialist. He had me keep a diary. Now that I recognize the symptoms and the phases, most of the time I can minimize the pain. Wish I knew this stuff twenty years ago."

—Jim M., Romeoville, IL

The awe of the aura
what are those lights?

One hallmark of migraine is the aura. About 20 percent of migraine patients experience auras, which follow the prodrome and last less than an hour. Researchers believe auras are caused by blood changes that then signal activity in the brain's cerebral cortex. The job of the cerebral cortex is to interpret information such as how we perceive sights, sounds, smells, and touch. Once this blood-flow change caused by the migraine reaches the cerebral cortex, the brain experiences glitches in its sensory abilities that result in the sensory disturbance known as the aura. Symptoms can be frightening, especially for those who experience the aura sporadically or for the very first time. Don't be afraid, though. The disturbance causes absolutely no permanent damage to your brain. (Do not fear that you are having a stroke.) In fact, many people function just fine while experiencing an aura. Though most clues are visual (blurry vision, flashing lights, or wavy lines), other sensory disturbances can be bizarre.

◆ Pins-and-needles tingling sensation or numbness of the face or the leg and arm on the side of the body where the headache generally develops.

◆ Difficulty finding words, speaking, completing thoughts; confusion.

◆ Vertigo (dizziness with a sensation of spinning). Some describe this symptom as a kind of hallucination of motion.

◆ Partial paralysis. (This is rare and temporary. But some people report paralysis of extremities, on the opposite side of the body where the headache is located, and of facial and eye muscles.)

◆Reduced sensation or a hypersensitivity to touch.

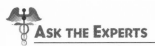

When my migraine comes on, I always see a bright small sphere with edges in the upper half of my vision. Are both my eyes being affected by this aura or is it only one eye?

Vision is actually a brain activity. The aura reflects a problem in the brain and this is projected as a visual disturbance of one side or another affecting the visual fields of both eyes. The aura does not localize to either eye, but to your vision. Think of the aura as an event, manufactured by your brain, that you "see."

Sometimes I see flashing lights that all but blind me. I am worried that these episodes will harm my eyesight. Does that ever happen?

No. Again, your eyes are not involved in the creation or viewing of the aura. It looks like you are seeing these blinding images, but they are not real and are not affecting your eyes.

Do medications for migraine affect the aura?

If the aura is your first clue that you are getting a migraine, and your treatment plan involves taking medicine to stop or abort your migraine, then that medicine should stop your aura too.

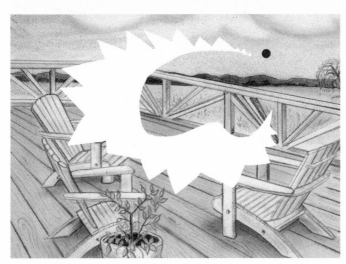

Auras are visual hallucinations that accompany 20 percent of migraines. There are all different types of auras, from dancing lights to partial loss of vision.

The big pain
the heart of the migraine

The headache phase, lasting from one hour to as long as three days, is the most debilitating part of a migraine episode. The pain is just one of the issues, however. Your whole body is involved. And yes, it's miserable. But again, knowing there is an end point to the pain is helpful—at least emotionally. Even better is recognizing early phases (so you might be able to forestall an episode) and making sure you are taking the right treatment—for you—during an episode.

◆ The pain is **hemicranial** (one side); can shift to the other side; or involve both sides, though this is less common.

◆ The pain, which can last from an hour to three days, gets worse with physical activity.

◆ Most migraine patients report that headaches begin in the early morning hours. In fact, many migraine patients find themselves with a headache upon waking.

◆ Aside from light- and sound-sensitivity, some migraine patients become nauseated; experience hot flashes or chills; feel dizzy and confused; suffer diarrhea or constipation; nasal congestion or a runny nose; and fluid retention or dehydration.

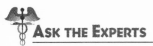

Aside from the head pain, I also feel very depressed whenever I get a migraine. Is that normal?

Yes, it is. Feeling apathetic and depressed or "out of sorts" are normal during a migraine. But those feelings resolve once the head pain is successfully treated. However, there is some research that suggests that having migraines may raise the risk of full-blown clinical depression. (The symptoms of depression include low energy, poor concentration, sleep disturbances, lack of interest in life, and suicidal thoughts. Depression should not be ignored—it requires prompt medical attention.)

I read that there is connection between depression and migraines. Is that true?

Depression may raise the risk of developing migraines. The apparent symbiotic relationship of the two disorders seems to suggest that depression and migraine may share some of the same biology, either relating to hormones or to neurotransmitters. Researchers who are studying this relationship recommend that people with one disorder be evaluated for the other. If you have migraines and are concerned about depression, talk to your doctor.

My migraines are pretty mild compared to what I have heard about them. Do I really have migraines?

Migraines cause a spectrum of pain, from very mild head pain to extremely severe head pain. If you and your doctor have discussed migraine and you fit the criteria and got a diagnosis, then the answer is "yes." Consider yourself lucky that you have a mild form of migraine. If you are not sure if your headache is due to migraine, then talk to your doctor and stay away from the trap of self-diagnosis.

The postdrome phase
the aftermath of a migraine

Though the headache pain has stopped, there is yet another phase to the migraine process, called the postdrome, or postheadache, phase. Most migraine patients take hours or even days to recover from the agonizing pain of the headache. Though some people report feeling "wrung out" or even experiencing a "major hangover feeling," it is unclear whether these symptoms are due to the migraine pain itself or to the medication the patient may have been taking.

After getting through the pain, some migraine patients report feeling depressed or simply being "low." They may also feel fatigued and unable to concentrate or comprehend information. These symptoms are temporary. How long the symptoms last is highly individualized. Generally, after a migraine has passed, a person is back to normal within one or two days.

Conversely, others report that they feel so euphoric after their migraine has passed that they can't believe how bad the pain was before. This up-and-down episodic nature of migraine is what keeps some people from seeking treatment.

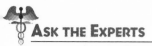

ASK THE EXPERTS

After a migraine, I always feel really rundown. My boss asked me point blank if I had a hangover. I was so upset, I didn't know what to say in response.

The resolution phase of the migraine is very draining. And yes, it can look as if you were hung over or have just gotten over the flu. Why not look at this as an opportunity to educate your boss about migraine. Many companies have established headache clinics as part of ongoing efforts to reduce the number of workdays lost due to migraine and other types of headaches and chronic illnesses. And some companies educate work-forces about available treatments. These educational efforts also help inform people without migraines or other types of "invisible" chronic problems. If you do decide to talk to your boss about your migraine, then see page 192. If you work for a large or medium-sized company, talk to the people in charge of employee health. Maybe they can hold a seminar. If you work for a small company—and are comfortable in the role—you might take time to educate your colleagues about the disease. Chances are good they know someone with migraines.

Types of migraine
which type do you have?

Your migraine may be somewhat different from the two most common types, migraine with aura or migraine without aura. Rather than lumping migraines into one broad category, specialists now look at migraines by various types. Though all share some basic features, there are several forms of the disease, and each person will suffer through the migraine in a very personalized way. Even if you usually experience the more common forms, you may, on occasion, experience another form of the disease. Some of these types of migraines may signal a new health problem that warrants more evaluation. That's why it's so important for you to always mention any unusual symptoms to your doctor.

The Headache-free Migraine

In this type, aura occurs without an actual headache. It only happens with individuals who have a history of migraine attacks.

Basilar Artery Migraine

This very rare form of migraine is accompanied by dizziness, vertigo, lack of balance, sleepiness, and confusion. It comes on suddenly and can result in fleeting visual disturbances, the inability to speak properly, ringing in the ears, and vomiting. Throbbing occurs in the back of the head. The basilar artery migraine is strongly related to hormonal influences and primarily strikes young adult women and adolescent girls.

Carotidynia Migraine

Also known as facial migraine, or lower-half headache, this type causes pain in the jaw and neck regions. Depending on the individual, the pain may be dull and aching or sharp and piercing and is often accompanied by tenderness of the carotid artery. This type of migraine is common in the elderly population.

Status Migraine

This type is characterized by long-lasting and severe pain. The pain often lasts more than three days. Hospitalization is often required.

Hemiplegic Migraine

If you suffer from this rare but severe type of migraine with aura, you probably also have a family history of it. The hemiplegic migraine often begins with neurological symptoms: paralysis and/or sensory disturbances on one side of the body, followed by the headache within the hour. People may also experience numbness or a pins-and-needles sensation. When the headache appears, the initial neurological symptoms may disappear.

Retinal Migraine

Another rare migraine, the retinal type, starts with a temporary, partial, or complete loss of vision in one eye. It is followed by a dull ache behind that eye that may spread to the rest of the head.

Abdominal Migraine

It's difficult to diagnose this migraine because the pain is felt in the abdomen. Nausea, vomiting, and diarrhea may occur, and the pain is usually in the middle of the abdomen. The attack typically lasts hours and occurs exclusively in children ages 10 and over. It is a forerunner to the migraine.

Helpful resources

Migraine: Pharmacology and Genetics
by Merton Sandler

Mechanism and Management of Headache
by James W. Lance,
Peter J. Goadsby

Migraine: Manifestations, Pathogenesis and Management (Contemporary Neurology Series)
by Robert A. Davidoff

Migraine: Winning the Fight of Your Life
by Charles Theisler

www.helioshealth.com/headaches

The National Foundation for the Treatment of Pain
www.paincare.org/migraine

CHAPTER 3

Treatment for Migraines

Goal-oriented treatment
migraines are as individual as you are

There is no reason to be in pain. Thanks to what science has learned about the migraine, the great majority of those with the disease can find relief by following a treatment plan that can include trigger avoidance, some lifestyle changes, and proper use of medicine. Some people may even be candidates for migraine prevention. A good migraine management program will include some very specific goals. You and your doctor should find ways to try to:

- Stop or reduce the frequency and/or severity of your attacks.

- Prevent migraines, especially if you have frequent migraines.

- Reduce any disability stemming from your attacks, such as missing work or social activities.

- Improve the quality of your life.

- Avoid rebound headaches, caused by medication overuse (See page 58.)

A good treatment plan will also include ongoing patient education that will help you manage your headaches. As you learn more about treatment, keep an open mind. Migraine is a chronic illness. And that means that no matter what marketers may say, there is no cure for this disease. Also, migraines are just as individual as you are. Drug regimens are generally based on what is most effective for the majority of people. So just because a drug works for your friend and not for you, doesn't mean you should give up hope. Let your doctor know how a treatment plan is working out.

Migraine drug treatment generally includes one or some combination of several classes of drugs, depending on the frequency and severity of your migraines and the degree of disability you experience. Unfortunately, these kinds of issues can be very subjective. That's why it is so important for you to keep your doctor updated regarding how well your treatment plan is working.

Classes of Migraines

Though anyone who gets migraines can experience many different types of attacks, from the extremely mild to the most severe, the majority of migraines fall into three distinct classes: mild, moderate. or severe.

A **mild migraine** means that it does not interfere with activity, such as going to work or to a social event—all the stuff of daily life.

A **moderate migraine** means that you may not be able to handle all your usual activities.

A **severe migraine** means that some activity is possible, but less than half of your normal activities are carried out. A disabling migraine is a form of severe migraine in which you must take to your bed, missing out on all activities, more than half of the time.

Aside from the severity of your migraines, your doctor will also look at other symptoms, such as nausea. If you experience this miserable symptom, ask about getting relief from your nausea.

One way for you and your doctor to gauge severity is through your headache diary or through a Migraine Disability Assessment Questionnaire, called MIDAS. MIDAS was created by Professor Richard Lipton of the Albert Einstein College of Medicine, New York, NY., and Dr. Walter ("Buzz") Stewart of the Johns Hopkins School of Public Health, Baltimore, MD, in partnership with AstraZeneca. Its goal is to help patients get the very best treatment when they see their doctors. It's only seven questions, and you'll get a score that ranks your migraine in terms of severity.

Migraine management
to mitigate, interrupt, or prevent?

Be thankful you're a 21st-century person with migraines. Otherwise, you might have wound up with a hole in your head. From ancient times through the 17th century, one of the most common ways to treat headache was a surgical procedure called trepanning, in which tiny holes were drilled in the skull to release evil spirits or noxious fumes, the presumed culprits behind the pain.

Though you may at times feel as if malevolent beings have taken up residence inside your head during a migraine episode, today's treatments are much more benign. No more holes in the head. No more live electric fish placed on the forehead, as was done at one time. And no more excessive use of narcotics that may have numbed the pain of a migraine but left most people who got migraines unable to function and suffering from rebound headache.

Today's treatments are many-layered. But they all boil down to two choices. Each choice usually requires different medications.

1. Taking medication to treat the pain of migraine. This is called "symptomatic" treatment. The medication can be over-the-counter, or prescription only. This includes taking medication (like the triptans) that *interrupt* the migraine process.

2. Taking medication to prevent the migraine from ever happening. This is called prophylactic or *preventive* treatment. (This is the option for people who do not respond to "symptomatic" treatment, or for those whose migraines are very severe or very frequent.)

Note: There are also nondrug treatments to improve your quality of life, whether you experience the most mild or most severe forms of migraine.

Drugs used to treat and prevent migraine

◆ Over-the-counter (OTC) drugs including acetaminophen or the non-steroidal anti-inflammatory (NSAIDs) medications like aspirin, ibuprofen, and naproxen.

◆ OTC combination medications that may include a blend of acetaminophen, aspirin, and caffeine.

◆ Prescription NSAIDs or prescription acetaminophen or combination drugs that include a sedative as well as acetaminophen, aspirin, and caffeine.

◆ Anti-nausea medication.

◆ Analgesics that can include aspirin or acetaminophen along with an opioid/narcotic medicine. Or a prescription opioid, like codeine, alone. (These drugs are considered "high-end" analgesics, are obviously prescription only, and are reserved for the most severe cases or for those who do not respond to other treatments.)

◆ Ergotamine and dihydroergotamine (DHE), work to reduce blood vessel dilation by contracting the smooth muscles including those in the blood vessels.

◆ Triptans reduce dilation of blood vessels. They are migraine-specific and work to interrupt the migraine process.

Preventing an Attack

These drugs are used to prevent migraines and are generally taken daily or once an attack has begun. They are best suited for those who experience frequent, severe, disabling migraines three or more times a month. However, there can be a case made for individuals whose migraines are less frequent, but equally disabling. There are several different kinds of medications.

◆ A class of drugs called beta-blockers or calcium channel blockers, usually prescribed for heart disease, can also reduce the frequency and severity of a migraine episode.

◆ Drugs used to treat epilepsy and bipolar disease called anticonvulsants have recently been approved for migraine prevention.

◆ Drugs that treat depression—specifically tricyclic antidepressants—may be appropriate for some patients. These drugs are thought to act differently on migraines.

◆ Anticonvulsant, drugs used to treat epilepsy and bipolar disease, are also used in migraine prevention.

Treating migraine pain
the medicines that can treat migraine

No two migraines are alike. Some come on quietly and build to a crescendo of debilitating pain; others come on quietly and leave you shaky but functioning. Finding the right medication to treat the pain takes time. Different people require different dosages of the same medication. Some require different delivery systems, be it pills, tablets that dissolve under your tongue, nasal sprays, shots, or suppositories. Some medications may be inappropriate for you because of your medical history. Here is a roundup of types of medications to treat the pain of migraine, but not prevent it from happening.

Analgesics to the rescue Chances are good that if you have experienced mild to moderate migraine pain, your very first stop was at your local drugstore or supermarket for some over-the-counter medications. You're not alone. It seems the majority of people with migraine rely on some over-the-counter help with pain. Whether it's aspirin, acetaminophen, ibuoprofen, naproxen, or some specially labeled over-the-counter migraine pain reliever, these drugs are probably your first line of defense, too. In fact, the FDA has approved certain over-the-counters like Excedrin Migraine, Advil Migraine, and Motrin Migraine Pain for use. Excedrin Migraine, which was the first to receive FDA approval, is actually a combination of aspirin, acetaminophen and caffeine. Caffeine is often added to analgesics because the caffeine improves absorption of the analgesic from the stomach. However, the caffeine may also interfere with sleep. Sometimes codeine and other narcotics are combined with analgesics.

The Ergotamines This class of prescription medications eases pain by reducing inflammation of brain nerves and constricting overly dilated blood vessels in the brain. (These drugs have fallen out of favor somewhat since triptans have been found to be more effective.) A cousin of the ergots called dihydroergotamine, or DHE, can stop a migraine in its tracks. It is available in nasal-spray form. But these drugs can cause drowsiness. They also can narrow coronary arteries and raise blood pressure, so they should not be used by anyone who has coronary artery disease. Check with your doctor before taking them. It may be that triptans (see pages 52, 164) would be more appropriate.

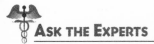

ASK THE EXPERTS

It feels like my skin hurts when I have a migraine. I know this sounds weird, but is it normal?

Absolutely. One study found that nearly 80 percent of patients experienced painful sensitivity to touch and temperature in specific areas of their skin. That may mean that migraine pain results from a kind of chain reaction along pain pathways leading to specific areas of the spine at the base of the neck. During the migraine process, nerve cells in the spinal cord may get stuck in an on position after they are turned on by certain chemicals. When the cells are stuck, even the slightest sensation—something like a blanket touching the skin, or hair brushing, for example—can be excruciating. The general term for this phenomenon is called allodynia.

Are some over-the-counters better than others?

Over-the-counter medications to help you with migraine pain generally depend on your preferences. Even the specially labeled over-the-counters (Advil Migraine, Excedrin Migraine, and Motrin Migraine) really aren't new drugs. They are just reformulations of existing over-the-counters in the same product line. The over-the-counter choice really is up to you. But remember, even though you don't need a doctor's prescription, let your doctor know what you are doing.

Interrupting a migraine
stopping it before it gets to be too much

Up until the 1990s, people who had migraines had few choices. They could take analgesics to help with the pain and ergotamines to blunt the force of a migraine. But it wasn't until Imitrex arrived on the scene in the early 1990s that migraine sufferers finally got a breakthrough medicine. Imitrex (its generic name is sumatriptan) is one of the first in a class of drugs called triptans that can stop a migraine once it has started.

How do triptans work? They mimic the action of the neurotransmitter serotonin whose job is to reduce the dilation of the surrounding blood vessels. Today, there are many triptans, all of which essentially work the same way, but there are some subtle differences. Also, the method of delivery of these medicines has improved. They can be taken by pill, injection, or as a nasal mist. Best of all, if one particular triptan doesn't work, you have a choice of others that might do the job. Similarly if one of the triptans has a particularly irksome side effect, another triptan may be just right.

These migraine-specific medications have been referred to as "miracle drugs", especially for those with moderate to severe migraines or those who have menstrual migraines (see Chapter 4). Triptans are termed abortive (stopping a migraine in progress) medications. They can't prevent the occurrence or frequency of migraines. They are used to stop the headache itself and the associated symptoms. And they are the fastest-acting of all drugs available, sometimes achieving pain relief in less than 30 minutes. You may not be a candidate for a triptan if you have uncontrolled high blood pressure, diabetes, are pregnant or breastfeeding, have high cholesterol, or have a family history of heart disease. On the plus side, many pain medications can be taken safely with a triptan.

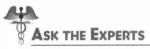

Ask the Experts

What side effects do triptans have?

The triptans do have a host of potential side effects, including flushing, neck pain, muscle tightness, difficulty concentrating, rash, tingling in the extremities, shortness of breath, sleepiness, a heavy feeling in the chest, and dizziness. However, though one triptan may cause you to feel short of breath, another may not. Some patients find that taking an **antinausea medication** such as belladona alkaloids complements the triptan. These drugs not only reduce or eliminate the nausea, but can also help a person relax.

What is the window of opportunity for taking a triptan?

In order to be effective, you need to take triptan medicine as soon as you feel your first migraine symptoms. If you wait longer, it may not be effective at stopping your migraine.

	Generic Name	**Brand Name**	**Potential Side Effects**
Triptans	Sumatriptan	Imitrex	Dry mouth, nausea, vomiting, dizziness, fatigue
	Zolmitriptan	Zomig	
	Naratriptan	Amerge	
	Rizatriptan	Maxalt	
	Eletriptan	Relpax	
	Frovatriptan	Frova	
	Almotriptan	Axert	

Preventing migraines
medication to stop them before they start

If treatment for the pain doesn't work for you, and triptans aren't stopping your migraines, or if you suffer from severe migraines or your headaches are too frequent, you and your doctor may want to plan a course of prevention with medication. Preventive drugs are generally taken daily. And, of course, they have side effects and are inappropriate for many patients. The decision to pursue a course of migraine prevention with drugs is usually reserved for the most severe cases and those that do not respond to other treatment. Here's a quick overview of some common drugs used in prevention. As with all other treatments, discuss this approach with your physician.

Beta-Blockers Typically used to treat certain heart problems, beta-blockers are often the first-choice drug for prevention of migraines. They work by affecting the response to nerve impulses in some parts of the body. You may need to take beta-blockers for several months before they are most effective. Examples of beta-blockers include inderal and tinolol. Side effects of beta-blockers may include fatigue, depression, impotence, dizziness, and exercise intolerance. This makes them problematic for athletes.

Calcium Channel Blockers These medicines used to treat cardiovascular problems can help with pain and help relieve aura symptoms. However, sometimes it can take weeks or months for benefits to be seen. The most prescribed drug in this class is verapamil. Side effects of calcium channel blockers include low blood pressure, headache, and constipation.

Antidepressants Although usually used to treat depression, tricyclic antidepressants can be effective in preventing migraines. Often, lower doses are used to treat migraines. Examples of tricyclic antidepressants include amitriptyline, nortriptyline, doxepin, and imipramine. Side effects of tricyclics may include drowsiness, dizziness, dry mouth, headache, sensitivity to sun, and weight gain. Another class of antidepressants are selective serotonin reuptake inhibitors (SSRIs). Examples include fluoxetine, sertraline, paroxitine, and fluvoxamine. Note: Some find the SSRIs are not as effective as the tricyclics for preventing headaches. Side effects may include anxiety, diarrhea, drowsiness, headache, nausea, trouble sleeping, and sexual dysfunction.

Nonsteroidal Anti-Inflammatory Drugs Regular, low-dose use of nonsteroidal anti-inflammatory drugs (NSAIDs) can be effective in preventing migraine headaches. These drugs work by reducing inflammation and swelling. Over-the-counter NSAIDs include aspirin, ibuprofen, and naproxen. Prescription-strength is also available. However, these medicines may have adverse effects when taken often over a long period of time. (See page 58.)

Anticonvulsants Several anticonvulsants that are used to treat seizures in those who have epilepsy have been found to prevent migraines, though the mechanism of action is unclear. These include gabapentin, valproic acid, topiramate and divalproex sodium. Side effects of these drugs vary but may include nausea, rash, hair loss, fatigue, weight gain, weight loss, and liver problems.

Ergot Derivatives Drugs containing ergotamine cause blood vessel constriction and often ease the pain of migraine headaches. These drugs come in several forms, including nasal sprays, tablets, injections, and rectal suppositories. Side effects of ergot derivatives may include nausea, numbness, dizziness, muscle cramps or weakness, and tingling. Patients who use these drugs long-term need to be closely monitored. There is a risk of dependency with some. Ergot derivatives can be toxic at high levels. (DHE has fewer side effects; it does not cause rebound headaches or dependency.)

Corticosteroids These drugs can help prevent headache pain by reducing inflammation and swelling. Prednisone is one example. Side effects with long-term use can include sodium retention, increased appetite, menstrual difficulties, and other problems.

Prevention medication primer
you have many choices

Many of the drugs used in migraine prevention were originally developed for medical conditions like high blood pressure, depression, and even seizures. Not all of these drugs have been specifically approved by the FDA for migraine prevention. However, because they have been approved for other conditions, doctors are able to prescribe these drugs "offlabel" for migraine treatment. For example, one new off-label treatment for migraine is Botox injections. (See pages 168–169.)

When these drugs are used for migraine prevention, the dosage is different than what you would receive if you received a diagnosis of clinical depression or heart disease, for example. And don't worry. Being prescribed a drug for depression does not mean that you have a clinical depression. Rather, it means that your doctor felt it was the most appropriate drug for you, based on your migraine history and other factors.

Preventive drugs are not magic. They will not prevent all episodes. However, they will make your migraine episodes less frequent and, ideally, less disabling. If you do get a migraine and are on a regimen of prevention, you will still be able to take other medications to relieve the pain.

Migraine Prevention Medication

	Generic Name	Brand Name	Potential Side Effects
Beta-Blockers	Inderal Timolol	Propranolol Blocadren	Dizziness, impotence, fatigue, depression
Tricyclic Anti-depressants	Amitriptyline Doxepin Imipramine Nortriptyline	Elavil Sinequan Tofranil Pamelor	Drowsiness, decreased libido, weight gain
SSRIs (Selective Serotonin Re- uptake Inhibitors	Fluvoxamine Fluoxetine Paroxetine	Luvox Prozac Paxil	Decreased libido, weight loss/gain
Calcium Channel Blockers	Verapamil	Calan SR (sustained release)	Constipation, hypotension
NSAIDs* (Nonsteroidal Anti-Inflammatory Drugs)	Ibuprofen Naproxen Naproxen Sodium	Numerous non prescription and prescription–strength brand names available	Gastrointestinal irritation, long-term use can harm kidneys
Corticosteroids	Prednisone	Prednisone	Irritability, swollen face, insomnia
Anticonvulsants	Divalproex Sodium Valproic acid Gabapentin Topiramate	Depakote, Depakote ER, Depakene Neurontin Topomax	Weight gain/loss, nausea, rash, liver problems

Note: This list represents only some of the more common drugs used in migraine prevention. Side effect may vary. If you have questions about your drug treatment regimen, talk to your doctor.

* Do not self-treat with daily doses of over-the-counter medication. The long-term use of NSAIDs must be discussed with your doctor.

The rebound headache
how to avoid a common problem

It's a cruel irony, but it turns out that the very first thing you reach for to help your headache pain may the the very thing that keeps it coming back again and again. Researchers have found that the overuse of simple over-the-counter analgesics, such as ibuprofen or acetaminophen, can result in more frequent headaches and a worsening of symptoms once the medicine has worn off. They call it the rebound headache, and it can occur when pain medicine to relieve or prevent migraines is taken too often.

Essentially what happens is that your brain develops a tolerance to a particular pain medication, meaning that the amount of pain medicine you once used to treat or prevent a migraine is no longer sufficient. It also means that when the medication begins to wear off, your headache returns. And it will be a doozy, with pain symptoms becoming more severe. You might also experience withdrawal symptoms—anything from anxiety to nausea to irritability. Sure, taking more of the drug will relieve the pain and accompanying symptoms—temporarily. But when the medication wears off, the pattern starts over again, with headaches getting increasingly worse.

These types of headaches can occur with simple nonprescription analgesics (the "one aspirin is good, but four is better" routine that we're all guilty of on occasion) as well as with prescription-strength analgesics. You should only be concerned about a rebound if you use these medications frequently. What is the solution? You need to reduce and perhaps eliminate the use of the offending drug. And you will feel worse before you feel better, with symptoms of withdrawal—anxiety, irritability—almost guaranteed. Don't worry—most doctors do prefer to taper you off the offender, rather than have you go cold turkey. Once the rebound problem is taken care of, the drugs will have a better chance of working.

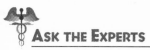

I heard that you can get a rebound effect from caffeine. Is that true?

Yes, the caffeine in your coffee, tea, or soda is a stimulant. It stimulates the heart and dilates the blood vessels in the body, while narrowing those in the brain. Moreover, it increases acid secretion in the stomach and acts as a mild diuretic or water pill. If you ingest caffeine on a regular basis, your body will get used to it and build up a tolerance for it. The day you forget that cup of coffee or tea, your body will feel the lack of its effect and respond with a rebound headache. There are 180 milligrams of caffeine in an 8-ounce cup of brewed coffee; 110 milligrams in an 8-ounce cup of tea; and up to 72 milligrams in a 12-ounce can of caffeinated soda. (Note: There are 15 milligrams in a 1-ounce piece of chocolate.)

My friend went to a doctor about her migraines, and she was immediately prescribed a triptan. My doctor told me to start off with some low-end analgesics for my migraine pain. What gives?

A lot may have to do with the differences between you and your friend's degree of migraine severity and frequency of episodes. It may also be due to the doctors's different approaches to care. Some doctors may prefer a "step" approach to care, meaning a doctor will begin treating pain with a lower-end medications for one or several episodes and then "step up" to other drugs if those lower-end products do not work. Others prefer a "stratified" approach to care, meaning the medication used is matched to the migraine severity. Learn more on page 62.

Managing without drugs
watching diet, sleep patterns, exercise, and stress

Though some type of medication is probably in your future, many people who get migraines report finding relief some of the time by following some very simple guidelines. Because they've kept a headache diary, they know their triggers. A smart plan for nondrug management of the disease means keeping an eye on your diet, sleep patterns, exercise, and stress levels.

Avoid your triggers

Avoiding your dietary triggers (see page 128) may be enough to offset some migraine episodes. Missing a meal can be a trigger, too. Keep to a regular meal schedule, all the time, even on weekends, holidays, and on vacation.

Drink water when exercising

Nothing is simple for people who get migraines—even exercise. For anyone who gets migraines, the dehydration that can come with exercise may provoke a migraine. If dehydration during exercise is a trigger for you, some studies show that adequate warm-up, hydration, and nutrition during an activity will help offset the headache. In any case, discuss exercise with your physician if you feel it is a trigger. And work out a plan that can keep you moving. Exercise has so many health benefits that turning into a couch potato is not an option.

Get your zzzzzzz's

Regular sleep patterns can also help offset the pain of the migraine. So try and keep a sleep routine, going to bed and waking at the same times every day, even on weekends and on vacation.

Chill out

Though stress migraine is not a stress-related disorder but an actual disease, it can trigger a headache as well as worsen one that is underway. When stressors become overwhelming, we all suffer the consequences, whether we get migraines or not. Relaxation techniques as simple as breathing exercises can help you better manage stress levels and maybe stop a migraine before it even starts. (See Chapter 11.)

FIRST PERSON INSIGHTS

Heaven is one headache a month

"Finding the right treatment for my migraine is really an ongoing process. I used to get migraines weekly, sometimes twice a week. Some medications worked for a while, then stopped, so my doctor and I kept trying new ones. For the past year, I've been on two medications, one to stop a migraine in process, and one to try and prevent the migraine. So far, so good. I'm down to about one headache a month, sometimes two. Compared to the way my life used to be, this is heaven. I can actually plan things with my friends and not worry about a migraine."

—Leryn D., Encino, CA

Your treatment plan
matching your medication to the pain

When you see your doctor about your migraine, be honest about your condition. If you miss work because of your head pain, let your doctor know. If you're missing out on fun activities with your friends and family, let your doctor know. Don't fudge the truth in your headache diary (see pages 16–17). The more honest you are, the better your chance of getting a treatment plan that is individualized for you and for your needs.

The simplest treatment plan is a "Step" approach to care, starting off with a non-specific treatment like aspirin or ibuprofen (one of its brand names is Advil). For some people who get migraines, an aspirin and a cup of coffee may be enough to offset the pain. Coffee is advised because the caffeine in coffee will speed the effect of the analgesic's pain relief. And the caffeine in coffee, tea, or soda is a migraine abortive agent. In fact, a lot of people unconsciously reach for a soda or a cup of coffee when they feel a headache coming on. (A note of caution here: Overuse of analgesic medications and caffeine, whether prescription or nonprescription strength, can lead to a daily headache, called the rebound headache. See page 58.)

If those simple nonspecific treatments don't do the trick, then you will "step-up" to different medications, maybe to prescription strength NSAIDs, or DHE, or even a triptan.

Another treatment approach calls for stratified care, which matches medication to your reported level of disability. If, for example, you consistently miss work because of your migraine, you may begin your course of treatment with a migraine-specific medication like a triptan. Or you may be a candidate for drugs used in migraine prevention.

Some studies show that analgesics can dull migraine pain; others show they aren't effective for the majority of people who get migraines. Then there's patient frustration: A recent study found that most patients with migraine spent more than three years seeing doctors and receiving at least five prescriptions before finally being given a migraine-specific medication. That seems neither cost-effective nor a good way to improve the quality of your life.

If your doctor wants to start you off on an inexpensive regimen of analgesics, whether prescription or nonprescription strength, arrange a follow-up visit within a few weeks either in person or over the phone to determine effectiveness. If the treatment is not working, don't let it drag on for months. Talk to your doctor. Here are some questions to ask when working out your treatment plan with your doctor:

♦ What are the various benefits and risks of this medication?

♦ How long will it take this medication to take effect?

♦ What are the side effects and how common are they?

♦ What happens if I mix this drug with an over-the-counter pain reliever or another prescribed medication?

♦ Should I take a triptan?

♦ Should I take antinausea medication?

Treatment guidelines
primary care doctors weigh in

The nation's two largest groups of primary care physicians have recently issued their first set of guidelines for the prevention and treatment of migraines. The guidelines, formulated by the American College of Physicians (ACP) and the American Academy of Family Physicians (AAFP), offer the first line of treatment in headache care.

Even though some experts feel the guidelines may be too conservative, this is great news for those with migraine. It means migraine is getting the serious attention it deserves, whether you have mild migraines or the most severe form of the disease. Here is what they recommended:

◆ Nonsteroidal, anti-inflammatory drugs (NSAIDs) should be the first line of treatment. Aspirin (not for kids), ibuprofen, naproxen sodium and a combination of acetaminophen, aspirin, and caffeine have been shown to be effective.

◆ If these drugs don't work, patients and physicians should move on to drugs specifically developed for migraines, such as triptans or DHE (dihydroergotamine) nasal spray. (The use of opioid—narcotic— medications is reserved for those who do not respond to other treatments.)

◆ People who have severe repeated migraines should be evaluated for possible preventive therapy. Generally, good candidates for preventive measures are patients who have two or more migraines that last three or more days each month, those who fail to respond to migraine treatment, and/or use medication more than twice a week, or have "uncommon" migraine conditions such as aura (visual sensations).

◆ People who get migraines should be actively involved in formulating their own treatment plan. And they should chart their headaches and identify and avoid triggers. (See pages 16–17 for tips on how to track your headaches.)

◆ If patients have nausea or vomiting, nonoral remedies should be tried first. Nausea and vomiting should also be treated directly.

Migraine Emergency

Should you need to go to the emergency room
Even with the best treatment plan, some people with migraine may have to seek emergency room treatment due to the duration or the severity of a particular episode. One way to avoid a future trip may be to have a "rescue" medication available. That's a drug that you will take if your current treatment fails to provide relief. But even with a "rescue" drug you may be one of those people with migraine who, at some point, require emergency treatment.

During the most severe migraine episodes, it may be difficult to explain your symptoms, let alone fill out forms that require your insurance information. The National Headache Foundation recently developed forms to expedite the process. The forms can be found and downloaded at **www.headaches.org**. Click on the Education Resource tab and you will find the form listed. Click on it and print it out. (In essence, the form asks you to rate the scale of your pain from 1 to 10 and to list any medications you are on and the dosage amount.)

The site also has a form for your doctor to fill out. The physician form includes information about your current migraine treatment plan as well as other medications you may be taking. But most important, it states that you are not a drug seeker or a substance abuser, and that your migraines are so severe that you may occasionally require emergency room treatment. It also contains a checklist of symptoms, among other pertinent information.

Helpful resources

*Drug Treatment of Migraine and
Other Headaches (Monographs in
Clinical Neuroscience, Vol 17)*
by Hans Christoph Diener (Editor)

Managing Your Headaches
by Mark W. Green M.D.,
Leah M. Green M.D.

*The Triptans: Novel Drugs for
Migraine (Frontiers in Headache
Research Series, 10)*
by Patrick Humphrey (Editor), et al

Women and Migraines

Hormones and headaches
estrogen's pivotal role

Welcome to the world of hormones and headaches, particularly the migraine. As if it weren't difficult enough with all those dietary, lifestyle, and environmental triggers, females who get migraines also have an additional trigger—tiny molecules called hormones. Estrogen seems to play a pivotal role in migraine episodes for some women. Estrogen is produced by the ovaries, and it's this female sex hormone that makes women, well, women. It's responsible for a woman's reproductive system and secondary female sex characteristics such as narrow shoulders and broad hips, breasts, hair patterns, and fat distribution. Estrogen, though, is also the hormone that seems to have a favorable effect on blood cholesterol and lipid levels, and it also seems to slow the progression of osteoporosis, a bone-thinning disorder.

Estrogens are secreted by the ovaries throughout a woman's reproductive years—the very time that migraine is most prevalent among females. Does this mean there is a cause and effect? Researchers aren't sure. Though there is a cascade of neurological events happening during the migraine, one of those neurological factors at play during what we'll call the menstrual migraine is the fluctuation of estrogen levels. Menstrual migraines may be caused by the precipitous drop in estrogen during the second half of the menstrual cycle, the luteal phase—the time between ovulation and menstruation.

Although 60 percent of women with migraine say their head pain is worse during menstruation, which is sometimes referred to as a menstrual–associated migraine, only an estimated 10 to 15 percent have what experts refer to as a true menstrual migraine (migraine that occurs almost exclusively during or right before bleeding begins).

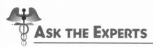

My migraines seem worse around my period. Do I have menstrual migraines?

Maybe. Doctors are not in agreement on the definition of menstrual migraines. If you're one of those women who note an increased number of headaches along with your menstrual period, you may not be considered by some to be a true menstrual migraine patient: a woman who gets a migraine around the time of her period—and at no other time. Some researchers believe "menstrual migraine" should only be used for women for whom 90 percent of all migraine episodes occur during the time of menstruation or a few days before. Call it what you will, but if your head pain seems to get worse around your cycle, discuss treatment options with your doctor, especially if you are taking birth control or hormone replacement therapy. (See pages 74–77.)

Are menstrual migraines really more severe?

It seems that way. A recent study conducted by Dutch researchers and published in the journal Cephalalgia showed that menstrual migraines tended to be more severe, of longer duration, and more resistant to treatment than migraines at other times of the month. About 60 percent of women with migraines experience an episode during menstruation. And even though just a small percentage of these women have what some experts call a true "menstrual migraine" the reality is the pain of the migraine can be exacerbated by nausea, cramping, backache, breast tenderness and bloating. Also, nonmigraine headaches around the menstrual cycle are very common.

Treating menstrual migraines
they may be different, but the treatment is not

Though menstrual migraines are predictable in occurrence, these headaches are treated in much the same way as other migraines: Drug therapy, trigger avoidance, and alternative approaches all seem to have a place. Most important, the same treatment rules apply whether you're a menstrual-migraine person or the plain-vanilla kind.

◆ Keep a headache journal. The headache journal (see pages 16–17) remains your most important tool. But if you find that your migraines are worse during your cycle, or you only have migraines during the time around your cycle, note that fact in your diary. Also, let your doctor know about other menstrual symptoms, such as severe cramping, heavy flow, and clotting, which may indicate other problems.

◆ Be an active participant in treatment. You are not a hormonal slave. Discuss treatment options with your doctor. Chances are good that something will work to alleviate your pain.

Generally, medication will include one of some form of the following drugs. They may sound familiar (see Chapter 3), but take a minute to review them. The list is not exhaustive.

Analgesics Nonsteroidal anti-inflammatories and combination analgesics containing aspirin, acetaminophen, and caffeine, and others.

Triptans For moderate to severely disabling menstrual migraines (See box, Triptans to the Rescue.)

Triptan Alternatives Ergots or ergot derivatives, along with antinausea medication, and a host of other drugs found in Chapter 3.

Triptans to the Rescue

Results from several large national studies show triptans can prevent menstrual migraines in as many as half of women who take them. One recent three-month study of the triptan frovatriptan recruited 545 women who had suffered from menstrual migraines for an average of 12 years. Starting two days before their period and continuing for six days, the patients were given either a placebo, a 2.5-milligram dose of frovatriptan, or a 5-milligram dose. Headaches disappeared in half those treated with the higher dose. Headaches stopped in more than a third of patients taking the lower dose, compared with about one-fourth taking placebo. Side effects including nausea, dizziness, headache, and fatigue were similar in all three groups.

A second trial enrolled about 450 women who had at least a one-year history of regular menstrual migraines. Within an hour after their headaches began, the women were given either a 100-milligram dose of sumatriptan, a 50-milligram dose, or a placebo. By one hour after treatment, almost one-third of women given 100 milligrams were pain free, as were about one-fourth of those given 50 milligrams. In contrast, 86 percent of women given placebo still complained of pain. By two hours later, about 60 percent treated with either dose of sumatriptan were able to go about their usual activities, compared with 36 percent of those taking placebo.

In yet another recent study of 290 women, naratriptan seemed to have a good effect on menstrual migraines, too. Compared with those on placebo, women who took naratriptan were more satisfied with its ability to control menstrual migraine headaches, either by preventing their occurrence or by reducing their numbers, severity, or duration. Just five percent of women reported drug-related side effects, such as nausea and fatigue, compared with three percent in the placebo group. And a recent large prospective placebo-controlled clinical study showed that zolmitriptan showed a higher rate of headache response at one, two, and four hours, compared to placebo in the treatment of acute attacks of "true" menstrual migraine.

Magnesium therapy
the mineral link

Women with menstrual migraine seem to have a high incidence of magnesium deficiency, which helps confirm a theory that magnesium is involved in the development of menstrual migraine. According to one study, during menstrual migraine, 45 percent of the women had a magnesium deficiency compared with 15 percent during nonmenstrual migraine and 14 percent during menstruation without migraine. Between menstruations and during times when there were no headaches, 15 percent of the women were found to have had a magnesium deficiency. (Although this theory isn't yet migraine gospel, some small studies have found that magnesium therapy could help reduce the frequency of menstrual-associated migraine. If you are looking to include more magnesium in your diet, good sources are legumes, whole grain cereals, and dark greens.)

FIRST PERSON INSIGHTS

Looking forward to menopause

"I really am one of those people who only get migraines around my period. I guess I'm pretty lucky, since I can control my headaches with just plain acetaminophen most of the time. About five times a year, I get really horrendous migraines about one day before or one day after my period starts. I do take a prescription medication at that time, so it's not that bad. But don't think it's that good either. I'm down for at least half a day, just wiped out. I still have about 20 years until I hit menopause. Maybe I'm strange, but I'm really looking forward to it."

—Gina M., Highland Park, IL

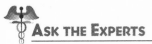
ASK THE EXPERTS

What about taking migraine medication if I am pregnant?

Most women who are pregnant try to avoid drugs—even women who get migraines with very severe headaches. These women hope they'll be one of the lucky ones whose migraines improve during pregnancy. But there may be a time when you must consider some use of medication, particularly if your migraines are so severe they cause nausea and dehydration, two symptoms that can be harmful to both you and the fetus if they are not promptly remedied.

The first thing you should do is talk to your doctor about your treatment plan during pregnancy. Many women turn to the nondrug approaches during pregnancy such as biofeedback, see page 144. If you have concerns about treatment and what you should do in case of a severe migraine episode, talk with your doctor about your options.

After I have the baby, can I go back on my medications and still breastfeed?

There are many advantages to both mother and child with breastfeeding. Some women delay the return of their cycle by breastfeeding exclusively, using no formula. For some of these women, their migraines do not return until the baby is no longer breastfeeding. Many medications are excreted in breast milk and can be passed on to the infant. Some medications, though, have very short half-lives. That means they don't stay in your system very long. Your best bet is to check with your pediatrician and your headache doctor for specific information about the medications to treat your migraine (or actually any medication you may be taking) and its effect on breast milk.

Hormonal therapy
stabilizing hormones may reduce migraines

One of the big questions facing scientists is whether oral contraceptives will help or harm women with migraines. Right now, the answer is not completely clear cut.

Some women who get migraines and begin taking oral contraceptives say their migraines become more frequent and more severe. Other women report that their migraines improve when they take a birth control pill. Yet others say their migraines began for the first time after taking the Pill.

These dramatically differing responses may be partly due to different formulations of oral contraceptives. When migraine begins for the first time following the use of oral contraceptives, it usually begins within the first few menstrual cycles. Rarely, however, do migraines begin after prolonged usage. But stopping the Pill may not result in immediate relief; some sufferers report that their headaches persist for up to a year; others report that these headaches cycles persist indefinitely. Women who experience migraine while on combination oral contraceptives (those that contain estrogen and progesterone) usually report that their attacks occur during the week that they are not taking the hormone.

By far, oral contraceptives are the most popular form of birth control. But as a woman with migraine, you must keep your doctor in the loop regarding how the Pill may be affecting your migraine frequency and severity. There are many birth control options available. Your best bet is to make sure the Pill is the right option for you.

Hormones as a treatment

Hormonal treatment for migraine is usually reserved for menstrual migraine that doesn't respond to traditional treatment. In theory, the use of hormones to help or even prevent migraine pain should work. Remember that stable low estrogen levels during menopause or stable high levels during the last two trimesters of pregnancy often diminish the frequency of migraines. Therefore women who get migraines should be able to be helped if their estrogen levels are stabilized, particularly if headaches have a hormonal trigger. In practice, however, the results of hormonal treatment are very unpredictable.

If you do not respond to traditional treatment, and if it is determined that you are a true menstrual migraine patient, your doctor *may* consider stabilizing your estrogen levels for brief periods of time. It's a big *may* and should be thoroughly discussed. Oral contraceptives have risks, as do any drugs. There are several approaches your doctor may try, perhaps reducing the frequency of your periods through hormonal manipulation or adjusting the dose of the oral contraceptive. The bottom line is that nothing is truly clear-cut about the use of hormones in migraine management. Sometimes it is a matter of trial and error. Other times, your doctor may deem hormonal manipulation entirely inappropriate for you because of specific health concerns or lifestyle issues such as smoking.

Risks of hormonal therapy
know the pros and cons

Though it would seem that women with migraines should never ever use the Pill, things aren't that simple. What you need to do is speak with your gynecologist and your headache doctor. There may be other forms of birth control that may be more advisable, depending on your risk factors. Or your doctors may find that a low-dose brand of oral contraception is okay for you. You should immediately contact your doctor if headaches do seem to get worse after starting a Pill regimen, or if the nature of the migraine changes.

Studies that have evaluated stroke risk in migraine patients are generally reassuring, however. There is some evidence that about 10 percent of women who get migraines and who experience the aura symptoms are at slightly elevated risk for stroke compared to those who get migraine without an aura, as well as those who do not experience the migraine. One study showed that women under the age of 45 with migraines, especially migraines with aura, had a three- to six-fold increase in stroke risk. If they smoked or used oral contraceptives (contraindicated for women smokers over 35), that risk jumped to about tenfold. That's a frightening statistic. However, it needs to be taken in context. Stroke is rare among young women. So an increased risk in a low number is still relatively low.

If you have concerns about stroke, the best thing you can do is quit smoking, eat well, control your blood pressure and your weight—essentially eliminate as many stroke risk factors as you can. Plus, if you have a family history of stroke or heart disease, take that as a warning that you need to be vigilant about controlling risk factors.

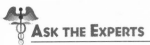

I'm approaching menopause. Should I even consider hormone replacement therapy since I get migraines?

Again, nothing is clear-cut about hormone replacement therapy (HRT) and the migraine, since HRT—the use of estrogen for women without ovaries or the use of estrogen and progesterone in women with intact ovaries—can exacerbate or improve migraine. However, remember that the majority of women do find relief from migraines once menopause hits. The peak age for females who get migraines is around 35 to 40. Some studies show that women who had a strong pattern of menstrually associated migraines are the very ones whose migraines tend to become less frequent and less severe as they age. This may be due to the fact that the hormonal trigger for younger women—that extreme drop in estrogen from previously high levels, a normal pattern before menstruation— starts to diminish. As hormone levels become constantly low in menopause, there is no longer a fluctuation and a drop in estrogen levels. That means the hormone-triggered migraines go away.

But on the flip side, in the general population of women over the ages of 55 to 60, the incidence of migraines is still higher than in males. So some factors other than hormones are at play. If you cannot take HRT or want to avoid it because of its well-reported risks, such as increased risk of developing breast cancer, there is some evidence that alternative treatments such as plant-based estrogens may be effective in treating hormonal symptoms like hot flashes. Other popular remedies include soy and kava. Some women find relief using an estrogen patch instead of pills, taking a synthetic estrogen, or adding testosterone to an HRT regimen.

The bottom line here is that there are real risks associated with long-term use of HRT. Inform your doctor of all of your medical conditions— especially the migraine—when considering hormonal manipulation.

Helpful resources

*The Hormone Headache: New Ways
to Prevent, Manage, and Treat
Migraines and Other Headaches*
by Seymour Diamond, et al.

*What Women Need to Know: From
Headaches to Heart Disease and
Everything in Between*
by Carol Colman, Marianne Legato

Migraine in Women
by E. Anne MacGregor

*The Women's Migraine Survival
Guide: The most complete, up-to-
date resource on the causes of your
migraine pain—and treatments for
real relief*
by Christina Peterson

Both of these sites are updated reg-
ularly and contain some good information on women and migraines, as
well as links to other sites.

www.achenet.org/women

**www.4woman.gov/faq/migraine.
htm**

Children and Migraines

Headache in children
it happens more than you think

Just like their parents, children and teens get headaches. In fact, research shows that more than half of all school-age children experience headaches. And an astounding 10 percent experience frequent, severe head pain that interferes with school, play, and other social activities. Before puberty, headaches affect both boys and girls with about the same frequency. But once the hormonal powder keg of puberty explodes at about age 12, girls are nearly three times more likely than boys to experience headaches, especially the migraine.

Of children with headaches, about 10 percent may experience migraines. But it's very difficult to get precise statistics regarding children and migraines, since youngsters—even teens—are often imprecise in telling doctors or their parents exactly how they are feeling. Like their grown-up counterparts, they need to learn how to pay attention to their bodies. (See pages 16–17.)

There are many reasons children experience headaches. Don't assume your child has migraines if she complains about head pain. Take a minute to review some of the most common types of pediatric headaches. Though some of the symptoms are surprisingly similar to those of migraine, don't fall into the trap of diagnosing migraine in your child. The same advice holds true for all people who get migraines, whether age 7, 17, or 70. Head pain needs an evaluation by a qualified medical professional.

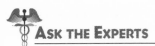

Do children get tension headaches?

For most children, headaches that occur only once are due to an infection (ear or sinus) or to a head trauma. For headaches that recur, tension or migraine is most likely the culprit. In fact, by age seven, nearly 40 percent of all children will experience a tension headache. Tension headaches usually hurt on both sides of the head, with a steady, non-throbbing pain that may feel like a pressure or tightness in the head. The child usually does not feel nauseated. Tension headaches last anywhere from a half hour to many days and, like migraines, can be exacerbated by stress. They used to be blamed on anything from peer pressure and school phobia to family problems and environmental factors, but no one really knows what causes them.

Are migraines hereditary?

Yes, migraine is an inherited disorder. If a parent has a history of migraines, then a child has a 50 percent chance of developing migraines. That percentage jumps to 75 percent if both parents have migraines.

Headaches in Children

If your child describes the headache as "the most awesome, worst headache of my life," or words similar to that, you should waste no time in getting her to an emergency room.

Migraine symptoms
they are different for children

When it comes to migraine, children are not little adults. Their symptoms are somewhat different. And, as with adults, migraine episodes differ among all children. Moreover, not every child with migraines will experience the same symptoms all of the time.

Generally, pediatric migraine symptoms include:

◆ Pain that is moderate to severe

◆ A feeling of throbbing or pounding pain

◆ A young child may have pain on both sides of the head, while an older child may only experience pain on one side of the head

◆ Nausea and vomiting

◆ Light sensitivity, scalp sensitivity, and "a sick feeling" from sounds or smells

If those symptoms sound familiar, that's because all mimic those of adults who get migraines. However, there are some marked differences for pediatric and adolescent migraine sufferers. In fact, the standard diagnostic criteria for migraine in adults only apply to 70 percent of children with migraines (see page 15).

Some of the differences:

◆ Headaches tend to last a shorter time (as little as an hour) in children.

◆ Migraine tends to occur in the front of the face and occurs on both sides in two-thirds of child patients.

◆ Children may often have a form of migraine known as a migraine equivalent or abdominal migraine, which does not cause a headache at all. Instead, children experience periodic bouts of nausea and vomiting (called cyclic vomiting syndrome) or other secondary symptoms found in adult migraine, such as a reaction against light or sound.

Migraine in children is disabling, as it is in adults. Migraine headaches may occur only once in a while or more than once a week. Between headaches, the child feels fine. In one study, children with migraine lost more school days than other children. Migraine triggers (see pages 88–89) in children are similar to those in adults, but anxiety, fear, and eating ice cream are also common triggers for children.

Children and the Aura

About 20 percent of children experience the "aura" before the head pain begins.Their aura is surprisingly similar to that of adult auras. Children experience the same flashing lights, spots, or zigzag vision— all aura benchmarks (see pages 36–37). However, symptoms in children also may include:

◆ impaired vision due to aura

◆ weakness in an arm or leg

◆ "funny" feelings like pins and needles in the extremities

◆ speech difficulty

◆ stomach aches

Headaches usually start during the aura or shortly after the aura stops. If your child complains of any of these symptoms for the first time, it is important to take him to a doctor. The doctor will make sure that the child is experiencing an aura (which does no permanent damage and goes away completely between headaches) and not anything more serious.

What the doctor needs to know
and what parents can do to help

If a child has frequent or severe headaches, he should be seen by a doctor. The same advice holds true for children as it does for adults: Make a separate appointment to discuss your child's headache. Do not tack on the phrase, "By the way, Johnny gets headaches," at the end of a routine pediatric visit. Childhood head pain—like adult head pain—needs a thorough evaluation.

The first step will be a careful medical history taken by your doctor. That involves the doctor asking you and your child questions that will help him understand why your child is having headaches. The doctor may ask questions about past illnesses or injury, when the child had his first headache and what her headaches have been like since then. These are the very same questions the doctor asks adults during a headache appointment. (See page 11.) The doctor will probably also ask the parents many questions about the child's recent headaches. And that's where the headache diary comes into play.

Your Child's Headache Journal

It will be difficult for a child to keep a headache journal alone. But it will be an important tool during the appointment. Consider the headache diary a kind of joint project. The information that's needed is similar to that for an adult patient. (See pages 16–17.) Information that you and your child can include:

- How frequent are the headaches?
- How severe are the headaches?
- At what age did the headaches begin?
- Does your child get headaches in the morning, afternoon, or evening?
- Does exercise (i.e., playtime) make the headache worse?
- Where is the pain located?

- Is it throbbing or constant?

- What does your child do when a headache occurs? Go outside and play, or retreat to a darkened room?

- Have you tried any treatments to help ease the pain? If so, what? Did it work?

- Does the pain awaken your child from sleep? Does the pain make it difficult for your child to get a good night's sleep or even take a nap?

- Do certain foods trigger a migraine?

- Has your child missed any school or social activities because of head pain?

- Do you or any other family member get severe headaches?

- And have you, the parent, received a diagnosis of migraine?

It's human nature to want to be with your child during a doctor's visit. But don't be surprised if you are asked to leave the exam room (or better yet, you could volunteer to leave, thereby making an instant ally of your doctor and possibly your child as well). Don't worry; you're not being asked to leave because you are annoying. But children can be very impressionable. Your doctor may want to ask your child these questions with you out of sight. Or if you and your child have completed a headache diary, the doctor may want to discuss the findings with your child. The reason? It's important for physicians to hear the child describe the symptoms in her own words. With adolescents, there may also be aspects of the headache that the child does not want her parent to hear.

Once a medical history has been performed, a doctor's visit may seem to go into overdrive. Migraine symptoms—actually any headache symptom in childhood—are often one of the benchmarks of more serious disease. And, obviously, it's very important to rule out these more serious conditions.

Getting a physical
checking for other problems

After the medical history, the doctor will perform a general physical exam. Vital signs will be taken, such as blood pressure and temperature. The doctor will also palpate (or touch with fingers) the head and neck looking for things like sinus tenderness, subtle soft tissue swelling that may indicate a goiter, and involuntary muscle spasms that limit neck movement. The doctor will also check for abnormal eye movement, problems with coordination, and other symptoms that may indicate a neurological problem. Don't be surprised if the circumference of your child's head is measured to see if it falls within a normal range to rule out intracranial pressure. Even your child's skin will be examined for abnormal findings.

All of these seemingly scary parts of the exam serve one purpose: to ensure your child's head pain is not due to a serious, underlying illness.

To Image or Not to Image

When it comes to children, the role of neuroimaging is rather controversial. Computed tomographic (CT) scanning or magnetic resonance imaging (MRI) is absolutely appropriate for pediatric patients with chronic-progressive headache patterns and those who have abnormal findings in the neurologic examination. But for the majority of children with normal findings, most doctors will not use high-tech imaging. That's because the overwhelming majority of research shows that it doesn't really add much to the diagnosis. However, there may be some instances when, even though your child is A-OK, except for those headaches, some high-tech imaging may be the next step. Here are some of the reasons your doctor may order some imaging tests:

◆ If there is loss of movement, sensation, or function, such as speech difficulty. These are called focal neurological deficits, and are caused by some kind of problem in the brain or nervous system.

- If the pattern of the headaches has gotten worse over time.

- If your child's optic nerve is swollen or if there are abnormal eye movements.

- If there are signs of meningitis, such as fever, stiff neck, rash, or stupor.

- If your child is younger than three years of age, and is showing any abnormal findings.

Art as a Diagnostic Tool

It's tough to talk to children about headaches. So researchers are using a new diagnostic tool: crayons. Think of it as Draw-A-Headache. Researchers found that among children with disabling headaches confirmed by both parental–and child-answered questionnaires, children's drawings about head pain not only helped doctors make a diagnosis more than 90 percent of the time, but also better defined how the headaches were affecting playtime and school. Some young people with migraines drew pictures of exploding heads, knives, jackhammers, and even high-heeled shoes sprouting from their noggins. Light sensitivity meant a lot of closed eyes, shut-off lamps, eyes covered with a blanket, and even a crossed-out sun. And, of course, there were lots of pictures of throwing up as well as spotty vision, pins and needles, and other symptoms of the aura.

When the diagnosis is migraine
helping to alleviate fear is the most important thing

A migraine diagnosis is good news. That means your child has no underlying life-threatening illness. That's not to downgrade a diagnosis of migraine. It is a serious, often debilitating disease. But there are treatments—for children as well as for adults—that can help minimize pain and even help prevent some future attacks.

Helping to alleviate fear is the most important thing a parent and doctor can do for a child with migraines. After all, even when you're eight years old and experiencing excruciating head pain, you want to know what is happening to you. Many doctors believe that explaining the migraine to a child—in a child's terms—is one of the most important therapeutic interventions that can be taken.

Children have fewer misconceptions about the meaning of a chronic disorder than do adults. Even though drugs may be vital in stopping the pain, a child understands the concept—and the importance—of altering lifestyle habits to help the headaches go away. And a child rarely likes to take medication, making childhood an ideal time to learn nondrug measures to cope with the migraine. Both you and your child's doctor can help your child understand that migraine is a controllable disorder with effective treatments.

Though doctors still don't know exactly what causes migraine headaches for adults or children, it's clear that triggers play an important role in the onset of the head pain for both. Children and adults share many of the same triggers (see pages 18–19), but children may have some special circumstances that can jumpstart a migraine.

◆ Stress. Though migraine is not a stress-related illness, stressors can trigger an episode. For children, upsetting events in school or home can prefigure an attack. Parents should ask children suffering from migraines if they are worried, upset, or anxious about anything. Stress for children usually originates at school or in the home. Any known stress, such as a recent divorce, change of school, even a parental job loss, should be discussed with the child's doctor.

◆ Hunger. In some children, missing meals or not eating enough at meals can trigger migraine headaches.

◆ Diet. Doctors think diet plays an important role in migraines for some children, though no one knows why. Foods that might trigger migraines are cheeses, chocolate, caffeine, citrus fruits, and food preservatives.

◆ Exercise. Hard exercise can bring about migraines in some children. Some research shows that eating before and after exercise may help prevent these attacks.

◆ Motion sickness. Children who experience motion sickness may later develop a migraine headache.

◆ Sleep deprivation. Not getting enough sleep or poor sleeping habits can trigger migraine headaches in children. Aside from obvious health benefits, good sleeping habits like going to bed and getting up at the same time every day may help in preventing a migraine episode.

Before banning any migraine dietary triggers, first determine if there is a link between certain foods and the headache. If a link is discovered, then it is time to talk to your child about the particular food. A dietitian may help you find substitutes. And your pediatrician can help you with education. Most children, once they understand a link between head pain and a food trigger, are more than willing to avoid that food in the future, especially if they are given other choices.

What about caffeine? If a child or adolescent consumes caffeinated soft drinks or several cups of coffee a day, it may be a contributing factor to the head pain. Caffeine abuse or withdrawal can precipitate or worsen headaches in adolescents. Remember, there's also hidden caffeine in some over-the-counter medications.

A personal treatment plan
tailor medication for home, school, and play

Before beginning any drug treatment, you and your child's doctor will first clarify the pattern, intensity, and nature of the migraine. A specific treatment plan has to be tailored to the patient's headache pattern, pain tolerance, and lifestyle. The daily use of preventive medications is also an option for pediatric patients with frequent migraines that interfere with their lifestyle. But the majority of young people who get migraines don't require daily preventive medications; they do need access to medications that can help at home, at school, and at play. Just like adults, children often need several rounds of trying different drugs before finding that magic solution, whether for an acute episode or for prevention. Each child is unique and will react differently to drugs.

Medication Choices

The following is a breakdown of some of the most common medications used to treat children and adolescents who get migraines. The list is by no means exhaustive. Remember, every child is an individual, and what works for another child may not work—or even be appropriate—for your child.

The absolute first-line of treatment is the occasional use of analgesic medication. Children seem to respond well to specially prepared pediatric liquid ibuprofen, as well as appropriate child doses of acetaminophen, ibuprofen, and naproxen sodium. Combination medications may also be helpful for some select patients.

None of the triptan agents are currently approved for use in children. There have been some extensive trials in adolescents using triptans that have demonstrated excellent safety profiles. If your child's migraine is moderate to severe and greatly affecting her quality of life, don't be surprised if your doctor suggests a triptan, depending on your child's age.

Unfortunately, nausea and vomiting occur in up to 90 percent of children with migraines. Many children will identify vomiting as the most disabling feature of a migraine. And vomiting can interfere with the effectiveness of oral medications. Antinausea drugs often give children a lot of relief, and some studies show that these classes of drugs alone can eliminate or reduce headache symptoms for some patients.

FIRST PERSON INSIGHTS

Chocolate was one of my triggers

"I had my first migraine when I was eight years old. I was in third grade and started crying and told the teacher my head felt bad and my eyes hurt. I remember that my dad had to come get me and take me home. When I got home, my mom started to cry. I thought I did something wrong, but then she told me she gets bad headaches, too. I was really scared. But it's okay now. I know about my migraines and my mom's, too. I had to give up chocolate, since my parents and I figured out that was one of my triggers. It's no big deal. I can have other stuff."

—Jeannine F., Boston, MA

Other strategies
your child has many options

If your child is missing school or other activities due to migraine and its associated symptoms, preventive medication may be considered. Studies show that many effective preventive medications prevent about 50 percent of migraines. But is it worthwhile to take a daily medication to prevent 50 percent of headaches? The decision needs serious evaluation. Generally, doctors will recommend prevention based on the frequency of attacks, the disabling nature of the attacks, and whether other treatment strategies are working. The recommended drug will be based on the child's age, medical history, and other factors.

Most commonly, the class of drugs chosen for migraine prevention among children and adolescents is consistent with that of adults: beta-blockers, anticonvulsants, and tricyclic antidepressants, among others. Cyprohep-tadine, an antihistamine, is often prescribed for migraine prevention in children because of its minimal side effects. Plus, it's easily tolerated by most children. But like adults, children and adolescents are faced with the same issues when it comes to prevention. These drugs do have side effects, and finding the right drug can be a process of trial and error. Prevention works for the majority of children who are deemed candidates for this approach, greatly improving the quality of their lives. The decision to undergo an often daily regimen of drugs, how long a course of prevention should last, and whether other nondrug approaches may be as helpful, are issues that need to be discussed with your child's doctor.

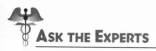

What else can I do to help my child?

There are many strategies you can employ to help your child. Most are really simple, and you are probably doing them anyway. Most doctors recommend that children who get migraines:

◆ keep regular bedtimes and regular wake-up times.

◆ eat meals at the same time every day.

◆ maintain a regular time for homework, and do homework in the same location.

But most important, doctors say that enjoying leisure activities should be at the top of the list—whether a child gets migraines or not. That means focus on the positive, rather than focusing on the migraine. The migraine should only be a small part of the overall identity of your child. And that's the same advice given to adults. How you get to that point, though, is really dependent on how well the migraine is managed. The good news is that most children really manage their migraines quite well.

I heard that biofeedback can help children. How does it work?

Children are very creative and open to suggestions. And some studies show that nondrug treatments, such as biofeedback and relaxation therapies, can be helpful, particularly in children These techniques can be taught to your child by a qualified professional. And then your child can try these strategies at home and use them to better manage—and sometimes even prevent—headache pain. (See Chapter 9)

Helpful resources

Headache and Your Child:
The Complete Guide to
Understanding and Treating
Migraine and other Headaches
in Children and Adolescents
by Seymour Diamond

Headaches in Children: Practical
Informative Guide for Parents,
Teachers and Paramedical Personnel
by Leonardo Garcia-Mendez

Coping with Migraines
and Other Headaches
by Andrea Votav

Headaches (My Health)
by Alvin Silverstein, et. al.

www.childneurology
foundation.org

www.pediatricneurology.com
Contains many resource links.

www.aap.org
The American Academy of
Pediatrics provides pertinent information on a variety of health topics
of interest to parents, from
headaches to nutrition to safety tips.

CHAPTER 6

Putting Together Your Team

Your primary care doctor
do you need another?

Your primary care doctor (also known as a family medicine specialist or internist) is probably the one who diagnosed your migraine in the first place. She was the one who picked up on your symptoms, spoke those words that you will always remember, and calmed your early fears about your treatment. This is the doctor who knows you best and, ideally, the one you want to help you care for your migraine.

She will chart your progress (including the records you keep in your headache journal), prescribe and make adjustments to your medicine, check for side effects and problems, and if problems arise, refer you to a specialist. Your migraine aside, you will still need your primary care provider nearby if you come down with other common ailments, such as an ear or sinus infection or the flu.

However, if none of the treatments prescribed by your primary care provider seem to work, and if migraine is not your only health problem—if you also have heart disease, for instance—you may want to be referred to a migraine specialist, though your primary care provider will still be in the loop, taking care of your other health needs.

Tips for Choosing a Primary Care Physician

If you move to a new town or take a new job with a different health insurance or HMO than your previous employer used, you will find yourself shopping for a new doctor to entrust with this crucial new factor in your life.

How to find a new doctor:

◆ Start with your former doctor. Chances are she will probably know someone to refer you to.

◆ Call the local hospital and see if it has a doctor on staff experienced in treating migraines.

◆ Call your local hospital's referral line. It will refer you to doctors in the area who are taking on new patients.

When you find a doctor who can treat your migraine, ask if you can do an initial interview to see if you're a good match. Ask before you go whether the physician charges a fee for this appointment.

Remember that under the Health Insurance Portability and Accountability Act that took effect in April of 2003, you have the right to a copy of your medical records. Before you switch doctors, get a copy and correct any errors. Make several duplicates to give to your new primary care physician and other doctors you may be seeing. Be sure to add the corrected records to your headache journal (see pages 16–17).

Neurologist
when your evaluation shows red flags

Primary care physicians are perfectly capable of treating migraine and, in fact, treat the majority of people who get migraines. However, some people who get migraines ask for a referral to a neurologist—a doctor who specializes in the treatment of nervous system disorders, such as strokes, headaches, dementia, and multiple sclerosis, among other diseases.

And in some cases, a neurologist may be called by your primary care doctor. Usually neurologists act as consultants to either make or confirm the diagnosis and to determine if further tests are needed and what treatment to consider. This neurological referral may be short term, meaning that once your particular situation is taken care of, you will be referred back to your primary care doctor. Or if your particular situation warrants, you may remain under the care of a neurologist and a multidisciplinary team of headache specialists who can help you find relief.

One of the main reasons for an immediate referral to a neurologist from a primary care doctor is the emergence of one or more of the following red flags during your initial evaluation.

◆ Your headache may be inconsistent with migraine.

◆ You may be experiencing a prolonged aura or one that is not typical.

◆ You have a complicated migraine type like basilar, or hemiplegic migraine (see pages 42–43).

◆ The diagnosis is not clearcut.

◆ You have another medical condition, such as coronary heart disease, that may complicate your migraine treatment.

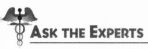

My primary care doctor has had me try a number of different medications for my migraines, but none of them are working. Will a neurologist help where he can't?

It depends. If you feel the treatment you are getting is ineffective, especially after several attempts with different types of medication, or if you are not receiving the respect and the time you deserve, it may be time to check out the specialists in your local hospital's department of neurology or at a headache clinic in your area.

My primary care doctor ordered an MRI of my head to rule out any other problems. Won't I see a neurologist to review my MRI results?

Not necessarily. Your results will be reviewed by a radiologist who may consult with a neurologist or neurosurgeon. If there are any unusual findings, then you will be referred to a neurologist. If everything is normal, then your primary care doctor will take it from there.

Ophthalmologist
catching eye problems early

Eye problems are rarely causes of migraine, or any headache, for that matter. But while you're making appointments, don't forget a yearly visit to see an eye doctor. If you can't seem to remember when you last had your checkup with an ophthalmologist, try using your birthday as a natural reminder. This appointment is especially important after the age of 45 when vision changes are experienced.

Ophthalmologists are physicians who can help you avoid and correct vision problems. When you arrive for your appointment, make sure to tell your doctor that you get migraines. Eye problems are rarely causes of migraine, or any headache, for that matter.

During your eye check, your doctor will look at the backs of your eyes for signs of eye disease, including early cataracts and glaucoma. See your eye doctor each year so you can be sure to catch any problems. If you do begin to deal with eye problems, your doctor might ask you to come in more often.

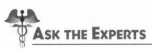

What is the difference between an ophthalmologist and an optometrist?

An ophthalmologist is a medical doctor who specializes in diseases of the eye. An optometrist is not a medical doctor, but someone who is trained to examine eyes for focusing defects and to correct them with glasses. An optometrist will look for signs of eye disease in a yearly exam. If she spots a problem, she will refer you to an ophthalmologist who will be able to medically treat your problem.

Are there any diseases of the eye that produce symptoms similar to those I experience with a migraine aura?

The visual disturbances that can accompany migraine can mimic other primary eye problems, such as retinal detachment and glaucoma, and neurological disorders, such as stroke and brain tumors. Migraine visual symptoms, however, are short lived; not so with these other diseases.

FIRST PERSON INSIGHTS

Backup shades

"I recently met with my eye doctor to get my routine check-up. An assistant dilated my eyes, and then the ophthalmologist checked my eyes. After 10 years of checkups, so far so good. The most irritating part is the paper-thin, squared off-disposable sunglasses they give you for driving home. Call me vain, but I feel ridiculous wearing them even on the ride back to my office. I always forget to bring sunglasses, but I finally got smart and now keep a cheap pair in my car so I won't forget."

—John F., College Park, MD

Your advocate
when you need emotional support

Migraine is tough to handle on your own. Simply managing this chronic illness calls for serious attention, enough to give you a case of chronic stress. You can reduce some of that stress by letting someone close to you help take some of the burden off your shoulders. That someone can be a close friend or family member—someone who understands you and cares deeply about your well being.

Consider asking your advocate for help with the following.

◆ Going in with you to your doctor appointments and perhaps bringing up a concern that you've forgotten to mention to your doctor.

◆ Preparing a healthy meal for you when you are suffering from head pain.

Other things your advocate can do.

◆ Exercise with you to lower stress and blood pressure.

◆ Pick up supplies at the pharmacy.

◆ Help with holiday shopping.

◆ Arrange for child care when necessary.

◆ Remind you of migraine triggers, such as alcohol, when you are tempted.

◆ Talk with you about things that are stressing you out.

◆ Share a good joke or movie.

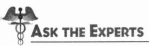

ASK THE EXPERTS

I don't want to burden my friends or family with my migraine. Are there mental health therapists who specialize in chronic illness?

Yes, there are. Many people can become overwhelmed with chronic illness, leading to depression and other issues. Many therapists focus their practices exclusively on these types of issues. However, any licensed mental health expert may be able to help you develop strategies for coping with anxiety or depression that is negatively affecting your health. It's hard to take care of your migraine when you're feeling overwhelmed. Some therapists lead support groups, and others meet one-on-one with migraine patients or with the patient and members of his family, since migraine can affect those around you.

Ever since my migraine diagnosis, my friend has not let me alone. I can use her help, but she goes overboard on everything. What can I do?

It sometimes happens that an overly helpful friend will take on your illness as her own crusade. You need to draw some boundaries around your situation. One way to deal with overeager helpers is to give them set tasks. This way they won't be tempted to take over everything. If the problem persists, tell her your concerns about her behavior. If that does not work, take a break from each other for a while.

How to be a smart patient
making the most of your appointment

The door opens up in the exam room, and the doctor enters and asks how you're doing. You draw a blank. All the ups and downs of the last few months seem distant and hard to remember. And it feels like the clock is ticking on your appointment.

To avoid this all-too-common situation, treat your appointment like a business meeting, complete with agenda, in this case, a list of your questions and concerns. How do you do this? Through preparation. Before your appointment, review your headache journal (see pages 16–17). Be sure your journal contains a log of your recent migraine episodes and full details about your day: what you ate, what you did, what time of day the pain started, and what you did to find relief. Think of your doctor as a health partner, so the more information you can provide, the better.

Have these ready on the day of your appointment:

◆ Copies of medical records from prior evaluations. (If this is a first visit with a new doctor, consider sending a copy of your medical history a week of so before your appointment.)

◆ A list of medication tried in the past and their benefits and side effects.

◆ A list of questions you have about your migraines. (Concentrate on your headaches and their associations; don't tack on questions about additional health issues.)

◆ A description of your current health problem. Try to keep it short and to the point. If you can, use medical terms. For example, "I have head pain lasting 4 to 14 hours, three times a month, consisting of right-sided throbbing pain, with extreme sensitivity to light and noise. I can't work at these times and take to my bed. This is more effective than "I have headaches."

Insurance Help

Insurance can be complicated and confusing, especially for people who need long-term treatment. It's not always clear what health services will be covered for migraine and other chronic disorders and for how long—or if you are prescribed a drug like triptan, how many pills are covered by insurance in a one-month period. Here are some tips that can help:

◆ Call ahead to your insurance company to determine what is and is not covered. Don't assume that insurance won't cover a particular service, such as dietary counseling or other types of referrals. If you have severe migraines that are affecting the quality of your life, see if you can get a preauthorized health service, such as sessions with a psychologist who can help with coping strategies.

◆ Work with your doctor to get letters of necessity to encourage your insurance company to cover a service that it initially rejected.

◆ Fill out claim forms fully; don't provide an excuse for a rejected claim.

◆ If a claim is initially rejected, appeal it.

Support groups
you're not alone

Support groups for migraine not only provide information and resources for people who get migraines, they also create a forum where members can share experiences and get support in a safe atmosphere. A support group can help you deal with the anxieties migraine sometimes brings on, such as changing roles for family members, feelings of lost control and fear, and the complications migraines cause. Other common issues discussed in support groups include dealing with a new diagnosis, having difficulty with a medication, avoiding migraine triggers, and general burnout.

Each support group has a facilitator who organizes the group and runs the meetings. Support groups are often led by a therapist, nurse, social worker, or by someone who also gets migraines. The facilitator can be helpful in making sure members' concerns are addressed and that medical information is accurate.

If you attend a support group, you'll likely learn about new treatments and ways to manage your migraine. You might learn about motivation techniques and how to maintain good control when you're having difficulty coping with your migraine. Here are two online support group sources:

www.migrainepage.com Ronda's Migraine Page is an excellent site and extremely active. It also offers continually updated links and information about migraine treatment, research, and regional support groups.

www.community.healingwell.com/community/?f=31 This is another very active site that offers information about migraine and a variety of diseases.

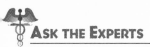
Where can I find a migraine support group in my town?

Go online. MAGNUM (**www.migraines.org**) hosts message boards. And it has a link to ACHE (American Council for Headache Education) that provides a state-by-state list of support groups. Or call your local hospital and ask about of any migraine support groups. They are often held in hospital meeting rooms, as well as libraries, parks, churches, and community centers.

What about online support groups?

There are a number of Internet lists and newsgroups that act as online support groups for migraine (see page 120). Online support groups work in a similar way to ones that meet in person—offering shared experiences, a calming voice for the newly diagnosed, and a way to reduce the stress of living with migraine.

I'd like to go to a support group meeting, but the idea of speaking in front of groups makes me nervous. What can I do?

This is completely understandable and absolutely common. Speak to the facilitator ahead of time and discuss your anxiety about attending a meeting. Bring a friend to the meeting if that makes it easier for you. Remember that a support group is designed to create a safe, comfortable space to share experiences and work through problems with people who are facing the same challenges as you.

Helpful resources

Heal Your Headache:
The 1-2-3 Program for
Taking Charge of Your Pain
by David Buchholz, Stephen
G. Reich

No More Headaches
No More Migraines
by Zuzana Bic

The Women's Migraine Survival
Guide: The Most Complete,
Up-To-Date Resource on the
Causes of Your Migraine Pain-
And Treatments for Real Relief
by Christina Peterson,
Christine Adamec

Migraine
by Oliver W. Sacks

Headache Help: A Complete Guide to
Understanding Headaches and the
Medications That Relieve Them
Fully revised and updated by
Susan Lang and Lawrence Robbins

The Chronic Illness Workbook
by Patricia Fennel

"In Bed," by Joan Didion,
from her book *The White Album*

www.migrainehelp.com
www.healingwell.com/migraines
Migraine Awareness Group, a
National Understanding for
Migraines (MAGNUM).

www.migraines.org
A national nonprofit group that acts
as a clearinghouse for information
about migraines.

CHAPTER 7

Using the Internet

Top migraine sites for laypeople
the best sites to start with

You have been given a diagnosis and perhaps even begun your treatment. If you are like most people, your first instinct is to find out everything there is to know about migraine. This is a useful instinct, so hold onto it. You don't need to become a migraine expert—your goal is to become an informed, active patient. After seeing their doctor, most people go home and turn on their computer and start in. You can too. But first, a word of advice—don't start by searching the main search engines such as AltaVista or Google, since these can overwhelm you with information. Instead, start with migraine-specific sites listed below to ground you in the basics about migraine. If you don't have Internet access at home, try your public library—many have Internet access stations that you can use for half an hour or more. The following sites provide comprehensive migraine information and are frequently updated.

MAGNUM—The Migraine Awareness Group
www.migraines.org

For anyone who gets migraines or who thinks they may be experiencing migraines, this should be the very first stop. The mission of this national organization is to dispel myths about the migraine and to improve the quality of life for those who get migraines. The site is very comprehensive, covering consumer-oriented research and treatment information, online forums, finding the right doctor, and much more. Because it is not overloaded with advertising, this site is easy to navigate.

The American Council for Headache Education
www.achnet.org

The American Council for Headache Education is a nonprofit patient-health professional partnership that promotes public awareness of headache as a biologically based illness. The information is first rate. The organization advocates individualized treatments, which combine the best of traditional medicine, alternative medicine, drug, and nondrug therapies.

The site offers support group information, online discussion forums, help in finding a qualified doctor, and a free newsletter.

The National Headache Foundation
www.headaches.org

Another nonprofit organization offering a wealth of information to people who get migraines. This well-organized site provides medical information as well as online support (including an e-mail pen pal program), a bookstore, and a continually updated list of ongoing clinical trials.

The Migraine Relief Center
www.migrainehelp.com

Though it is sponsored by a pharmaceutical company (GlaxoSmithKline), the information contained in this site does not push the use of such prescription drugs as triptans. The information is clear and concise. Its online resource library provides links to comprehensive migraine information, too.

General migraine health sites
when you want basic information

Discovery TV's Health Pages
www.discoveryhealth.com

An extraordinarily well-done health site that encompasses a host of diseases and disorders. A keyword search with "headache" produces a wealth of information on everything from a primer on head pain to migraine in children. All content is hyperlinked to other articles of interest.

Go Ask Alice!
www.goaskalice.columbia.edu/

Columbia University's Internet question-and-answer site. This site is supported by a team of Columbia University health educators and health care providers, along with information and research specialists from health-related organizations worldwide. Questions are archived so that you can review previous posts. And according to site information, all questions are read. The site offers its own search engine. Go Ask Alice! receives more than 1,500 questions weekly from college and high school students, parents, teachers, professionals, and older adults on every conceivable health topic. A keyword search using "migraine" and "headache" provides answers to a variety of questions, from the latest in migraine treatment to the connection between migraine and hormones.

Mayo Clinic
www.mayoclinic.com

Information from the Mayo Clinic is provided by Mayo Clinic physicians and staff. The award-winning site contains up-to-the-minute information on migraine, from self-treatment with over-the-counter medication to the transformed migraine (also called evolved migraine, a disorder in which a person has headache pain at least four hours a day on most days over a long period, possibly associated with frequent use of over-the-counter pain medicines). Other links include a drug search and tips for healthy living. The site also provides online health management tools and an opportunity to keep yourself updated on the latest news about your health condition. Registration is free.

HealthScout
www.healthscout.com

This general consumer health site provides a compendium of information from search engines like Yahoo! to consumer publications like *USA Today*. The site also contains the HealthScout encyclopedia, which can help you navigate through some unfamiliar terminology.

About—Migraine
www.headaches.about.com/mbody.htm

An extraordinarily well-done, well-documented site about the migraine, offering research and treatment news, links, chats, and discussions. The site is huge but extremely user-friendly. There is some significant advertising, but it is not insurmountable. If you don't want to read a pop-up ad, click the X in the pop-up box. Whatever information you may be looking for, this is a great place to start.

Smart Searching Tips

Put quote marks around phrases (as in "migraine aura"), and most search engines will exclude results that include isolated uses of each of the words. Also, if you put a minus sign in front of words appearing in the irrelevant results, you'll lose the words you don't want.

Top medical research sites
go to these for clinical information

Once you've got a basic grounding about your migraine, you'll be ready for something more substantial.

eMedicine
www.emedicine.com

This site promises "Instant Access to the Minds of Medicine." And that's exactly what you'll get with a compendium of up-to-the-minute journal articles. Registration is required. But it's free. Simply do a keyword search with "migraine."

National Institutes of Health's Medline
www.nlm.nih.gov/medlineplus/

This is the prime source for patient and professional information. Registration is free, and with it you'll have access to full-text and abstract information about the latest research and treatment information on migraine. Do not be put off by the titles of the articles. Take the time necessary to glean what information you can. And better yet, take a study with you to your doctor to get input on the information you've uncovered.

MedEm
www.medem.com

This site offers patients a host of information from leading medical societies, including the American Medical Association. Its medical library (use keyword search) provides full-text articles on the latest in migraine research and treatment. An excellent stop. Plus, if your doctor is a member of MedEm, you may be able to get some online consulting. Check it out.

The National Institute of Neurological Disorders and Stroke
www.nunds.nih.gov

This is a textbook example of a well-documented Web site that contains both consumer- and physician-oriented information, research abstracts translated into plain English, and numerous, easy-to-navigate links providing more in-depth information in bite-size chunks. Though some of the information is quite involved, the material is presented in a consumer-friendly manner.

The American Medical Association
www.ama-assn.org

American Academy of Family Physicians
www.familydoctor.org

American Academy of Neurology
www.aan.com

Again, all you need is the keyword search of "migraine" to find doctor-approved articles on migraine care, research, and treatment. These are in-depth sites that are continually updated and offer a mix of patient and professional information. Don't be afraid to access the physician information. You can get through it.

Medline Plus Health Information
www.medlineplus.gov/

This service is provided by the National Library of Medicine and the National Institutes of Health. A great resource for new research. The site offers a medical dictionary, drug information, and a medical encyclopedia.

The Merck Manual of Diagnosis and Therapy, Section 14, Chapt. 168
www.merck.com/pubs/mmanual/section14/chapter168/168b.htm

This huge pharmaceutical company manual provides a comprehensive view of migraine written for a nonconsumer audience. That does not mean it is not worthwhile. The overview is very good. Plus, by doing a search on the home page (**www.merck.com**) you will find a wealth of information on migraine, from drugs used to treat the disease to current research news.

Alternative approaches
looking outside the mainstream

If you're interested in learning more about various alternative therapies for migraine, your first stop should be those organizations that take an out-of-the-mainstream approach to treatment of various diseases.

The Alternative Medicine Foundation
www.amfoundation.org/

This site provides a primer on almost all forms of alternative treatment, including acupuncture, herbs, mind/body techniques, homeopathy, massage, and more. Much of the information contained on the site is free to the public, though there are some fee-based links.

American Holistic Health Organization
www.ahha.org

Feature articles, referral lists, and self-help information are the hallmarks of this site, which acts as a national clearinghouse for all things alternative. A great site to help you get associated with nontraditional approaches to care.

The National Center for Complementary and Alternative Medicine
www.nccam.nih.gov/

This government-sponsored site supports research on complementary and alternative medicine and helps demystify the alternatives by explaining which treatments work, which ones do not, and why. This site provides comprehensive information on alternative approaches integrated into traditional practices. Well worth your surfing time.

Holistic-Online
www.holisticonline.com

This site offers a compendium of alternative approaches to treatment of various diseases. The migraine-specific pages include in-depth information on coping and preventive approaches using alternative treatments.

There are a wealth of other sites that you can peruse by simply keying in "migraine and alternative treatments" in a search engine. Many of the sites contain interesting and useful information. However, some are laden with advertising promoting special products, such as vitamins or herbs. Before you buy anything, make sure you talk to your primary care doctor. There is a lot of snake oil for sale, and most of it can be found on the Internet. Check out Quack Watch at **www.quackwatch.com**. This organization keeps tabs on fringe alternative therapies.

Doctors and Internet-Savvy Patients

Not too long ago, many doctors scoffed at the idea that the Internet would make patients more informed. After all, the doctors were the experts. Times certainly have changed. In fact, most doctors today are used to patients gathering information on the Net, and then presenting that information during an office visit. In fact, some doctors grudgingly admit their patients may actually be as well informed as they are about specific treatments for some disorders. Doctors, too, use the Net to research and read the latest news and to communicate with peers. That makes the Internet the Great Equalizer. The key to being a savvy patient, though, is the way that you present your Internet findings to your doctor. Tossing a bunch of printouts on your doctor's desk isn't the best idea. Instead, if you are interested in a particular treatment, say Botox for migraines (see pages 168–169), bring a printout of several studies with you. That way you can keep a discussion on point.

Surfing for a specialist
using the Web to find a migraine specialist in your area

Without a doubt, the best way to find a doctor is through a referral from another physician, a medical specialty organization, a medical center in your region, or even from a family member or friend with migraines. However, you can use the Internet to aid your search—especially if you are looking for a second opinion or want to change physicians. Many doctor-finder sites also offer health insurance information. Choosing the right doctor often involves several visits until you find a physician who makes you comfortable and whom you trust. See Chapter 6 for more on building your medical support team.

At **www.doctordirectory.com**, you can find a neurologist, internist, or family practice physician by state and by region. The American Medical Association Web page, **www.ama-assn.org**, also provides a listing of general practitioners by state and by region. At **www.familydoctor.org**, the American Academy of Family Physicians also provides a doctor finder by region. As do neurologists: **www.aan.com/public/find.cfm**. In fact, almost all specialty sites offer ways for you to connect to a physician. Another way to find a doctor is to search for "headache clinic" within your city or region.

Also, don't forget to do a simple search of practitioner listings at the Web sites of the major hospitals within your city. Migraine-specific sites also offer doctor finders. For starters, try **www.migraines.org/help/helpclin.htm**, provided by the Migraine Awareness Group. This search engine will help you find clinics and specialists in your region who are approved by other people who get migraines.

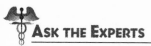

ASK THE EXPERTS

How can I keep a handle on all these great sites I am finding?

Bookmark them. This is a special file you create of favorite Internet sites. When you want to go to them, you simply click on your bookmark file and look through the list of your favorite sites. Click on the one you want and the Web opens to that site. How do you bookmark a site? While you are in the site you want to bookmark, go up to the Bookmark tab or Favorites tab or Favorite Places tab, and it will ask you if you want to add the site to your bookmark list. Click OK. You're done.

Online support
welcome to a world of where everyone has migraines

Often, the best person to talk to about migraine-coping strategies or the effect the disease has on family life or work, is someone who has experienced migraines. And that's where the Internet has proven to be a real blessing. Note: The best sites are monitored, meaning that behind the Internet curtain, there is a real person overseeing the site to ensure that online discussions stay focused and respectful. Some of the best sites include:

Ronda's Migraine Page **www.migrainepage.com**, is an excellent site and extremely active. It also offers continually updated links and information about migraine treatment, research, and regional support groups.

Another active site that offers information about migraine and a variety of diseases is **www.community.healingwell.com/community/?f=31**.

Both of these sites have received numerous accolades from health organizations. There is a wealth of chat rooms, forums, and message boards available to you. You might also try newsgroups, where you can ask questions, pick up advice (their e-mails are stored online for you to browse), and post your own so that others may benefit. One such popular site is **www.alt. support. headaches.migraines**.

By this time, your printer is probably breaking under the strain of all the pages of information you have been printing out. You don't have to print the entire article or even the whole page. You may just want to print bits and pieces. If so, just drag your computer mouse across the paragraph(s) that interest you so they are highlighted. Then go up to the File tab and click on Print. A dialogue box will open. Click on the word Selection. Then click on the OK button and you'll have a printout of the material you highlighted. Add these vital bits of information to your headache journal. Or if you wish, create a separate notebook just for your Internet research. Keep things simple, though. A three-hole punch will help you keep everything in a binder. Get some dividers so you can categorize your findings by topic.

FIRST PERSON INSIGHTS

The ribbing was worth it

"I use the Internet a lot to find health information. My family laughed at me because I was convinced that I had every disease that I read about. There was a point where I thought I had diabetes, sleep apnea, and monthly headaches. And I used to laugh at people who were such hypochondriacs! It's easy to get into a state of information overload. I did. The trick is to take the information to your doctor. I didn't have diabetes or sleep apnea. But I took a checklist of migraine symptoms that I found on the Net to my doctor. Turns out my monthly headaches are actually migraines triggered by my period. I never knew there was a connection between the two, and I had never mentioned the problem to my doctor before. My doctor has me on medicine that helps ease the head pain considerably. Thanks to the Internet, I am pain free. So, all of the ribbing I got from my friends and family was actually worth it."

—Jeannie S., Detroit, MI

Evaluating a Web site
all Internet sites are not created equal

The Internet can be a fabulous source of information, giving us the power to reach out and consult experts all over the world. It can also cause sleepless nights if you find information that frightens or harms you. There are many tales of people who inflicted great harm to themselves by self-diagnosing and self-treating after reading information on the Internet. And there are many tales of how the Internet has helped patients and doctors in diagnosing a rare ailment and finding the best treatment. To avoid the pitfalls and to make the most of the Internet, follow these simple guidelines:

◆ Don't rely on one or two sites for all of your information. Seek information from multiple sources, especially those institutions that you trust.

◆ Having hundreds of links on a site doesn't automatically ensure accuracy. Anyone can link to multiple sites. And those links don't represent endorsement.

◆ Medicine changes quickly. Check the date of the content. You may actually still find sites that say that migraine is not a disease, or that it is purely vascular in nature.

◆ There is no such thing as Internet diagnosis. If someone says he can diagnose your migraine over the Internet, move on. And make an in-person appointment with your family doctor.

◆ If you do share medical information with an expert over the Internet (you may if you use discussion forums or Q&A capabilities on some sites), make sure that information is kept confidential or "cloaked" to ensure privacy. Check the site's policy to make sure your private information, such as your name and phone number, is not sold to a third party.

◆ The first thing you should do when surfing through a site is to find out who sponsors the site. You want information from qualified specialists: medical doctors, licensed practitioners, medical associations, local and national hospitals, and organizations of a reputable nature. Sites sponsored by such specialists are credible, since they are primarily focused on providing top-notch information.

◆ Make sure it's complementary. Any credible site will state that the information contained in the site is not a substitute for a medical evaluation. Be wary of sites that tell you their way is the best approach to migraine treatment.

◆ Look for the seal of approval. Web sites that post the Health on the Net Foundation's (HON) code of conduct are monitored for their compliance to a code of ethical conduct. Check **www.hon.ch/HONcode/ Conduct.html**.

◆ Follow the money. Don't be put off by the ads you may see on some credible sites. Use common sense. If a site is pushing a particular drug, a miracle cure, or an approach to treatment that just seems wrong, move on.

Don't Forget Your Local Library

Have a library card? If the answer is yes, you have access to databases through your local institution's Web site. Almost all major libraries offer database links. All you need is a library card with a valid number that you will then type in to get access to the database. There are hundreds of databases you can use to access up-to-the minute news articles and full-text research papers about migraine. One of the easiest-to-use databases is InfoTrac, generally available free of charge to library patrons.

Helpful resources

After Any Diagnosis
by Carol Svec

The Health Resource
www.theheathresource.com
Tel: 800 949-0090
You don't have to search the Internet yourself.
There are a number of companies that offer this
service for a fee. One such company, called The
Health Resource, will do extensive Internet
research complilation that is customized to your
diagnosis. The company's Internet specialists
will then comb through the Internet and other
sources and locate medical articles geared
toward your specific situation, including mainstream, experimental, and alternative treatments
along with top specialists. In a week to 10 days,
you will receive a hard copy of their findings in a
bound booklet, complete with glossary. Prices
range from $150 to $400.

The Role of Nutrition

Food fundamentals
what does food have to do with headaches? plenty

Earlier in this book, you learned that headaches result from a complex
cascade of events that produce blood vessel changes that alter blood flow.
Among the numerous contributors to blood vessel changes are stress, elevated levels of compounds like glucose in the blood, neurotransmitters like
serotonin, and diseases that are accompanied by blood vessel damage,
including heart disease and diabetes. So what does food have to do with
headaches? Plenty.

Blood vessels respond to stress and other triggers by either narrowing
or widening. Some of these triggers are food-related. For example, eating
carbohydrates stimulates the body to produce serotonin, a stress-related
neurotransmitter that causes brain blood vessels to dilate after they've
tightened up from a stressful situation. The compound tyramine, found in
yogurt, nuts, and lima beans, causes blood vessels to constrict and can lead
to migraines in people who are susceptible to this type of headache. Lack of
food, too, can lead to a migraine from low blood sugar or dehydration.
Conversely, following a diet that improves the health of your blood vessels—
for example, a diet to help treat heart disease or high blood pressure, can
alleviate your headaches. The food-migraine link can be a powerful one.

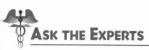

ASK THE EXPERTS

Whom should I hire to help me figure out what to eat?

The best person to hire is a registered dietitian (R.D.). Registered dietitians teach you about the basics of healthful eating and about making specific changes in your diet to help treat your migraines.

What's the difference between a nutritionist and a registered dietitian?

A nutritionist has studied nutrition and often has a master's degree. Registered dietitians are health professionals who have completed an accredited education and training program and who have passed a national credentialing exam. Many registered dietitians also have master's degrees in nutrition.

How do I find a dietitian?

You can find a dietitian on your own through the Yellow Pages, by contacting the American Dietetic Association at **www.eatright.org** or 800 877-1600, ext. 5000 for names of dietitians in your area, or by asking your insurance carrier for names of approved providers. Also be sure to ask your doctor for names of dietitians that he or she recommends for patients with migraines or conditions that may contribute to migraines.

What happens when I see a registered dietitian?

At your first appointment, a registered dietitian will review your medical history, ask you questions about your current diet, and plan changes to your eating habits that are appropriate for your illness. At follow-up appointments your progress will be reviewed and your diet adjusted as needed. Consultation with an R.D. for medical purposes is covered by some insurance plans, but not all, so check with your insurance company regarding your coverage.

Trigger foods

you can't shun them all, but you can avoid the major ones

Trigger foods are foods that can spark a migraine headache because they contain compounds that cause arteries to constrict or dilate in susceptible individuals. One such compound is tyramine, which is derived from the protein amino acid tyrosine. Aged cheeses such as cheddar and parmesan contain high amounts of tyramine. Migraines also can be triggered by other compounds derived from amino acids: monosodium glutamate, used as a flavor enhancer in Asian and prepared packaged foods; phenylethylamine, in chocolate; and aspartame, in artificial sweeteners. Nitrites (found in salted, cured meats, salt-pickled foods, and smoked foods) and sulfites (preservatives in wine, dried fruit, baked goods, condiments, and some soy products) trigger migraines in some people. You may be susceptible to one or more of these compounds.

Medications can react with food components to cause migraines. One type of antidepressant medication, a rarely used MAO (monoamine oxidase) inhibitor, constricts blood vessels and dramatically increases blood pressure if foods with tyramine are not cut out of the diet. Warnings about the interaction between medications and foods appear on the written material that comes with prescription drugs.

While it is impractical and virtually impossible to eliminate every possible trigger food from your diet, you can keep a food diary and follow an elimination diet to weed out major culprits.

Common Trigger Foods

Type	Food
Alcoholic beverages	Red wine, vermouth, champagne, beer
Beverages with caffeine	Coffee, tea, caffeinated soft drinks
Dairy products	Aged cheeses, such as cheddar, Parmesan, blue cheese
Breads	Sourdough, breads made with fresh yeast
Vegetables and fruits	Some types of beans (broad, Italian, lima, lentil, fava, soy), sauerkraut, peas, avocados, overripe bananas, dried fruit (apricots, figs, raisins)
Meats	Salted and cured meats (ham, corned beef, sausage, bacon, lunch meats), dried meats, pickled herring, chicken livers
Nuts	Peanuts, peanut butter
Soups	Canned and from dry mixes (if containing MSG)
Sweets	Chocolate
Seasonings and additives	Monosodium glutamate (MSG), sodium nitrite, soy sauce, marinades, meat tenderizers, aspartame

Caffeine and alcohol
they have opposite effects

You enjoyed dinner out, with several drinks and glasses of wine, and then had a leisurely cup of espresso. You decide to sleep in, but instead of feeling better, you wake up with a whopping headache. You may not have realized that both caffeine and alcohol have strong ties to headaches.

When you drink a beverage with caffeine—coffee, tea, cola, some non-cola sodas, and energy drinks—the blood vessels in your brain constrict. Too much caffeine—say, three or four cups of coffee—over a short period may cause headaches in some people. Caffeine can also cause sleeplessness and rebound headaches that come back every day. More common is the headache you get from caffeine withdrawal if you wait too long for that first cup of coffee. Without caffeine, your brain's blood vessels dilate, or widen, changing the speed of blood flow and causing your head to pound. The best remedies are over-the-counter pain relievers or more caffeine.

Alcohol has the opposite effect. It dilates blood vessels, as well as irritates them. A hangover headache is not caused by alcohol itself, but rather by the dehydration and low blood sugar that can result from drinking alcohol. Additionally, some alcoholic beverages, namely red wine, contain headache-causing natural compounds called congeners. The best migraine remedy is prevention. Here are some tips:

◆ If you consume caffeine, do so at about the same time every day to prevent withdrawal symptoms. Try to cut back to one cup a day, or better yet, none at all. And no soda.

◆ If you drink alcoholic beverages, drink in moderation and have at least one cup of water or nonalcoholic beverage between alcoholic drinks.

◆ Drink alcohol only after you have eaten; food helps slow the absorption of alcohol.

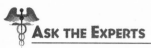

Will I get a headache from drinking energy drinks?

Energy drinks typically contain about the same amount of caffeine as a
cup of coffee, along with additional herbal caffeine-like stimulants. This
combination can cause caffeine-withdrawal headaches and headaches
from dehydration, especially if you mix energy drinks with alcohol.

How can I kick the caffeine habit without getting bad headaches?

Slowly cut down on the amount of caffeine in your day by mixing regular
coffee or tea with decaf, first half regular, half decaf for a couple of days,
then one-quarter regular and three-quarters decaf. At the same time,
switch to caffeine-free soft drinks. After a few more days, cut out all caffeine. Even this way, you still may get a headache.

Why do many over-the-counter headache medications contain caffeine?

Because of caffeine's effect on brain blood vessels, it can help relieve
headaches, but taken over a period of time, it can actually worsen them.
If you're trying to avoid caffeine, read labels carefully and avoid brands
with caffeine—many say "extra strength."

the elimination diet
finding your food triggers one by one

Can't figure out what is causing your headaches? You may want to try an elimination diet. Start by eliminating all possible migraine-causing foods and beverages listed below. Wait a few days. Then, one by one, add back foods or groups of foods, say, cheeses, and keep a food diary to record any reactions. Wait at least two days before adding new foods to your diet. Strict elimination diets are not balanced nutritionally and should not be followed for long periods of time.

Here is a list of foods and additives to cut out:

Alcohol and Vinegar

Red wine, champagne, beer, dark-colored liquors; balsamic or red wine-vinegar

Aspartame (Nutrasweet)

Bread Products

Fresh-baked, yeast-risen bread products

Caffeine-Containing Beverages and Foods

Regular coffee, tea, iced tea, and cola; caffeine-containing soft drinks; chocolate

Dairy Products

All cheeses except American, cream, and cottage cheese; cheese-containing foods, such as pizza; yogurt, sour cream

Fruits

Citrus fruits (orange, grapefruit, lemon, lime) and their juices; raisins and other dried fruit; bananas, red plums, canned figs, avocados.

Monosodium Glutamate (MSG)

Chinese food; many snack foods and prepared foods; hydrolyzed vegetable/soy/plant protein; natural flavorings; yeast extract; many soups, broths, stocks

Nuts and Peanut Butter

All nuts and nut butters, including peanut butter

Processed Meats

Hot dogs, sausage, bacon, salami, bologna and other meats that are aged, canned, cured, marinated, tenderized, or contain nitrates or nitrites

Vegetables

Broad, lima, fava, and navy beans; pea pods, sauerkraut, onions

A food journal is essential for figuring out which foods, if any, are contributing to your headaches. You don't need to buy a notebook—instead, make your own journal pages by hand, or on the computer. Keep them simple and easy to carry with you during the day. Maintain your food diary for at least a week and for as long as you are working with the elimination diet and reintroduction of foods.

Each journal page should have room for the following columns:

◆ Date

◆ Meal and time of day

◆ What you ate and drank, being as specific as possible and including cooking method and condiments

◆ How much you ate

◆ What you were doing while eating

◆ Your mood, paying particular attention to stress or anxiety level

◆ Headache, if any, and time it developed

Discuss your findings and discoveries with your physician, who may refer you to a registered dietitian for guidance and diet advice.

Improving the odds
tweak your diet to help keep migraines away

A well-balanced diet, minus any foods that give you headaches, is the best diet for migraine sufferers. You'll get all the vitamins, minerals, and nutrients you need for good health. You can tweak your diet, however, to improve your odds for keeping migraines at bay:

Try eating less fat and more carbohydrates. Researchers at Loma Linda University in California found that a diet high in complex carbohydrates—whole grain bread, cereals, grains—and lower in fat reduced the frequency, intensity, and duration of migraine headaches.

Include foods with the mineral magnesium, which may help reduce the frequency of migraines. Foods rich in magnesium include nuts, fish, dried beans and peas (kidney beans, lentils, split peas, and others), bran flake cereal, and dark green, leafy vegetables like spinach and kale.

Eat smaller meals more frequently, up to six times a day, to help keep blood sugar steady. Allowing more than four or so hours between meals can cause blood sugar to drop and the blood vessels in your head to dilate, leading to headaches.

Drink plenty of caffeine-free, nonalcoholic beverages to ward off dehydration and its headaches.

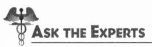

ASK THE EXPERTS

How do I avoid getting a headache when I'm overly hungry?

The sensation of hunger is metabolically complex. You should keep hydrated and eat often. In general, you should allow no more than four hours to pass between meals and snacks in order to help keep your blood sugar steady.

What should I eat to prevent low blood sugar?

Avoid meals and snacks that are mostly processed carbohydrate, like pretzels, cookies, candy, or juice, because they are absorbed extremely quickly and can cause your blood sugar to rise sharply and then drop down equally fast. By adding a protein to a carbohydrate snack, you will keep your blood glucose levels on a more even keel because the protein will slow down the absorption of the carbohydrate. Choose meals and snacks with a carbohydrate and protein, for example, apple slices and peanut butter or whole grain cereal with milk. Also, it's a good idea to eat whole grain, unprocessed carbohydrate foods, such as whole cereals, crackers, rice, and bread—they are absorbed more slowly than processed grain foods.

Eating for your health
the fundamentals are simple

Healthy eating is right for everyone. But what is healthy eating? If you follow news headlines, you may be confused about how to eat right. High protein or high carbohydrate? Low fat or high fat? Unlimited fruit or no fruit? Cut through the clutter, however, and you'll find that the fundamentals of healthy eating are quite simple.

Portion size

Proper serving size is most important to healthy eating. Many of us eat portions that are too big and supply too many calories. To start, review our guide to serving size, modified from the U.S. Department of Agriculture's Food Guide Pyramid. Portion sizes of packaged, take-out, and restaurant foods are too big and filled with too many calories. It's no wonder that more and more people are overweight! A simple guide to portions can help you retrain your eyes and stomach toward smaller servings; use measuring cups and spoons for more exact guidance. A registered dietitian or weight management program can offer you an individualized eating plan.

What to eat

The USDA Pyramid recommends a range of servings per day from each food group. If you are trying to lose weight, start with the lowest number of servings recommended.

Include grain foods like bread, cereal, pasta, and rice

Why: Your body needs these grain foods for their carbohydrates, the body's top energy source. Grains also supply important minerals and B vitamins. To get enough fiber, choose whole grains whenever possible; for example, a whole grain cereal at breakfast and for lunch a sandwich made on whole wheat bread.

Budget: 6 to 11 servings daily (each meal may have more than one serving)

Guide to serving size:

Food	Serving Size	Common Measure
Bagel	1/2 small	1/2 packaged English muffin
Bread, toast	1 slice	Slice from standard loaf
Breakfast cereal (cold)	1 cup	Standard teacup
Pasta or rice	1/2 cup cooked	Cupped palm

Enjoy fruits and vegetables.

Why: Fruits and vegetables dish up vitamins A and C, fiber, and a slew of natural compounds that are good for overall health. They also are filling and relatively low in calories.

Budget: 2 to 4 servings of fruit; 3 to 5 servings, or even more, of vegetables

Guide to serving size:

Food	Serving Size	Common Measure
Fruit	1 medium	Baseball
Fruit juice	6 fluid ounces	Juice glass
Vegetables	1/2 cup	Bulb part of light bulb

Eating for your health, cont'd.

Bone up on dairy products.

Why: Dairy products like milk and yogurt supply calcium, the mineral necessary to build strong bones. Calcium is particularly important for those at high risk of osteoporosis—older women and people with hyperthyroidism. Cheese also supplies calcium but is higher in fat and calories. To control calories, choose reduced-fat cheese, along with low fat or nonfat milk and yogurt. Try calcium-fortified juice or soy milk if you do not use dairy products.

Budget: 2-3 servings

Guide to serving size:

Food	Serving Size	Common Measure
Cheese	1 ounce	2 dominos
Milk, yogurt	1 cup	Standard yogurt container
Fortified juice, fortified soy milk	1 cup	Standard yogurt container

Include a variety of proteins.

Why: Meat, poultry, fish, beans, eggs, and nuts all supply protein, the nutrient your body needs to build and repair muscle and tissues. Each also offers its own unique benefits; for example, meat is high in iron and zinc, fish supplies omega-3 fatty acids, and beans have fiber. The Food Guide Pyramid recommends relatively small portions.

Budget: 2 servings daily

Guide to serving size:

Food	Serving Size	Common Measure
Beans (kidney, pinto, etc.)	1/2 cup (replaces 1 oz. meat)	Bulb part of light bulb
Eggs	1 (replaces 1 oz. meat)	Large egg
Meat, chicken, fish	3 ounces	Palm of a woman's hand
Peanut butter	2 tablespoons	Size of 1 walnut

Limit extras.

Why: Foods high in fat and sweets, like snack foods and desserts, add calories without a lot of nutrients.

Budget: Only occasionally

Guide to serving size:

Food	Serving Size
Butter, margarine	1 teaspoon
Chips, snack foods	1 ounce (about 1/2 cup)
Salad dressing	1 tablespoon
Sugar	1 teaspoon

Helpful resources

American Dietetic Association
Complete Food and Nutrition Guide
(2nd Edition)
by Roberta Larson Duyff, M.S.,
R.D., C.F.C.S., American Dietetic
Association
Sound advice on eating, including
chapters on nutrition and health
conditions and dietary supplements.

The Headache Prevention Cookbook:
Eating Right to Prevent Migraines
and Other Headaches
David R. Marks, M.D.,
and Laura Marks
Guidelines for following an elimination diet, also with recipes excluding
potential trigger foods.

Headache: Hope Through Research
www.pueblo.gsa.gov/cic_text/hea
lth/headache/head1.htm
The Federal Citizen Information
Center provides an overview of
headaches in general and migraines
specifically.

National Institute of Neurological
Disorders and Stroke
www.ninds.nih.gov
Web site of the government's agency
handling biomedical research on the
brain and nervous system.

American Dietetic Association
Tel: 800 877-1600
www.eatright.org
Offers nutrition information,
including consumer tips, fact sheets,
FAQs, resources, and referrals to
dietitians.

National Headache Foundation
Tel: 888 NHF-5552
www.headaches.org
A nonprofit organization dedicated
to educating headache sufferers and
health care professionals about
headache causes and treatments.

National Migraine Association
Tel: 703 739-9384
www.migraines.org
Offers comprehensive and up-to-
date information on migraines.

Complementary Therapies

Stress management
teaching your mind to soothe your body

You can cope with your migraine and feel better by using techniques to slow your heart rate, help you stay calm, and reduce blood pressure. Everyone benefits from learning how to deal with stress—even those with mild migraine pain. Practitioners of the so-called mind-body modalities teach you to be more conscious of stress and give you practical things to do about it. It may seem counterintuitive to focus on stress; after all, we're hardwired to recoil from pain and culturally programmed to roll up our sleeves and get on with things. But with proper guidance, stress management techniques can yield enormous benefits, not just physically, but also mentally, emotionally, and spiritually. **Relaxation therapy** encompasses a wide range of techniques designed to reduce stress and tension. Some of the more popular ones are:

Progressive muscle relaxation You do this by systematically tensing and relaxing the muscles in each part of your body. While sitting comfortably or lying down, inhale and clench your facial muscles, hold the tension for a moment, then exhale and relax those muscles. Do the same thing with your shoulders, one arm, then the other, and so on through your body until you get to your toes. When you're done, stay quietly where you are, and breathe normally for a few minutes.

Guided imagery The idea here is to imagine a peaceful place, and put yourself in the scene. This is usually done with a partner who provides the "guidance" by describing the scene, but you can do all the imagining yourself, or listen to a narrated audiotape or soothing music or environmental sounds, such as birdsong or ocean waves.

Diaphragmatic breathing Taking a few minutes each day to practice slow, deep breathing can relieve muscle pain, light-headedness, and improve mental acuity. All you need to do is stand, sit, or lie still; slowly inhale until you feel your lungs are full; then exhale slowly and completely. Repeat that for ten or twelve breaths, and try to do it from time to time throughout the day. Some people find it energizing to do this type of deep breathing before they get out of bed in the morning.

Biofeedback
learning to control the pain

Biofeedback is one of the most effective therapies not only for migraines but also for the stress of many chronic conditions. And because of its success, many experts don't even consider biofeedback an "alternative approach." It is an integrated component of their treatment plans. The National Institutes of Health considers biofeedback to be mainstream medicine and recommends its greater utilization.

Biofeedback works on the principle that you can be taught to control certain body processes that essentially seem to happen on their own, like heart rate, skin temperature, or even brain waves. To get the information—the feedback—that will allow you to learn to change the way your mind/body responds to stress and pain, such as blood-vessel dilation and muscle tension—the biofeedback practitioner uses small sensors, usually placed on the hands, shoulders or scalp. These sensors are connected to a computer. Depending on which sensors are attached, the computer will transform the information it receives and make it visible or audible via the monitor or speakers. This allows you to see or hear your breath rate, pulse rate, skin temperature and conductance, even your brain waves, live and in color!

You will then be taught how to breathe more deeply or be asked to visualize a relaxing scene, which will actually influence the sensor readings and thus what you hear or see via the computer. During a training session, you will practice various relaxation techniques while getting continuous feedback from the sensors. Thus, you can see how relaxed breathing can lower your pulse rate or change your brain waves. And you will see how sensitive your body is to stressful thinking. After several sessions, you will be able to consciously exert greater control over your mind/body responses, and see and feel the changes as your hands warm, your muscles relax, your breath slows and deepens, and your mind relaxes.

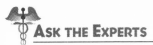

Why are sensors placed on the hands?

Skin temperature and skin conductance are usually measured on the fingers. The sweat glands and the blood flow through the hands are especially sensitive to stress and emotional reactivity. The stress response lowers peripheral blood flow which makes hands and feet feel cold, thus the expression "getting cold feet." When you learn how to profoundly relax, your hand temperature will rise and skin conductance will drop. Over time you can learn to sustain a lower level of stress and reactivity throughout the day.

How do you teach your brain to change its waves?

The basic principle in all biofeedback is that once you can perceive something you can begin to change it. The computer makes your brainwaves appear before you, linked to a graph or to a game like a maze. At the beginning of the maze is a blinking light. If your brain is producing the selected brainwaves, you can power that blinking light to race through the maze. The blinking stops when your brain moves out of the selected zone of brainwave output and starts again when it gets back into the zone. Depending on which brainwaves are being trained up or down, this method can help people learn how to focus their thinking, and can lower tension throughout the body, which in turn results in fewer headaches.

Where can I find a biofeedback practitioner?

The best place to look is the Internet. Check out the Biofeedback Certification of America at **www. bcia.org** or the Association for Applied Psychophysiology & Biofeedback at **www.aapb.org**. Both sites have tabs to help you find a practitioner in your area.

Meditation
using the metaphysical to help the physical

Studies show that regular meditation can lower blood pressure, relieve chronic pain, and reduce cortisol levels, a measure of the body's stress. It may also help if you suffer from frequent and severe headaches, and can help teach your body how to relax. Dr. Herbert Benson, a Harvard cardiologist, did a great deal of research on meditation and found that regular meditation can actually lower autonomic nervous system activity—meaning that meditation allows your body to truly relax. Dr. Benson dubbed this phenomenon the relaxation response.

How can something as simple as meditation perform such wonders? There is no hard answer. Most practitioners say it works because it transports both the body and the mind into a uniquely unified state. As meditation teacher Dr. Lawrence Edwards explains, "Meditation is a transformation process. Over time, meditation evolves into a process where you feel a sense of peace and inner freedom. Every time you meditate you are increasing the reservoir of meditative power that you can tap into during stressful or challenging moments."

There are a number of different meditation techniques to consider. Some focus on the breath, requiring you to simply observe yourself breathing in and out; others use a mantra (a sacred word or phrase) that is repeated over and over again. The goal is the same: to focus your attention away from the thoughts whirling around inside your head. The repetition of breath or mantra helps calm the mind so it can enter into a meditative state. Unlike guided imagery (see page 142), classic meditation does not involve talking or music, but it may be helpful to light a scented candle or burn incense. That's because your mind will associate the fragrance with relaxation, registering that it's time to settle down, and that can help ease your transition. It's also helpful to meditate at the same time every day and for the same amount of time, even if it's only for a few minutes.

How to Meditate

Find a place where you can sit quietly without interruption for 20 minutes.

Sit comfortably, but keep your back erect—this will help support alertness and open breathing. (You can meditate lying down if you are not able to sit up.)

Set a timer for 15 to 20 minutes.

Close your eyes and bring your attention to your breathing. Focus on the movement of your diaphragm as you inhale and exhale.

As you settle into this quiet breathing, you can silently repeat your mantra or any word you wish. You can use the traditional Sanskrit words *om namah shivaya.* or silently say a phrase of your own choosing, or simply use the words "one, two, three, four."

When your mind begins to wander, as it inevitably will, just gently return your focus to your breath or mantra. This pattern of wandering and returning is the beginning of teaching your mind to let go of its worries.

When the timer buzzes, notice how peaceful you feel.

Open your eyes and stretch.

Chose a regular time and place to meditate. Start by meditating for 20 minutes three times a week. Stay with it.

The complementary approach
look before you leap

Twenty years ago, if you mentioned to your doctor that you were pursuing
biofeedback for migraines, you might as well have said you were looking for
a psychic healer. But patient demand has since dictated that medicine
become less high-tech and more high-touch—and the use of nontraditional
treatments, has steadily risen. In fact, today, even the prestigious National
Institutes of Health has recognized the trend with its National Center for
Complementary and Alternative Medicine. Among its goals are to find out
what treatments actually do provide relief for various diseases. According to
an article published in the April 2003 issue of the journal *Neurology,* more
than 30 percent of headache patients, including migraine patients, do not
respond (or at least do not respond enough) to traditional pharmacological
treatments. That's why more patients—and their doctors—are looking at
the alternatives with a critical eye to determine what works and what
doesn't.

When used alone, these out-of-the-mainstream treatments are often
referred to as alternative. When used in addition to conventional medicine,
they are often referred to as complementary. According to the National
Institutes of Health, the list of what are considered to be complementary or
alternative therapies changes continually as they are proven to be safe and
effective and become adopted into conventional health care, and as new
approaches to health care emerge.

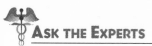

Ask the Experts

Where do I find alternative practitioners?

The National Center for Complementary and Alternative Medicine suggests that you contact a professional organization for the type of practitioner you are seeking. Often, these professional organizations provide referrals to practitioners as well as information about the therapy. Professional organizations can be located by searching the Internet or directories in libraries (ask the librarian). One directory is the Directory of Health Organizations Online (DIRLINE), compiled by the National Library of Medicine (**http://dirline.nlm.nih.gov**). It contains locations and descriptive information about a variety of alternative health organizations.

What happens if my doctor says no to anything alternative?

First, most physicians are recognizing that their patients often seek alternative treatments without informing them. Your doctor will probably be happy that you are even discussing the concept before you plunge ahead. If your doctor says no, without giving you a reason other than that she thinks it's all a "bunch of baloney," you will have to weigh her position against your desire to try something new that may or may not help your migraines and might even harm you. It also depends on what treatment you are seeking. Some of it is baloney, some of it isn't. Chances are good, though, that your physician will respect your desire for a remedy, regardless of where it comes from. Whatever you do, be sure to keep your doctor informed.

What to expect

identifying your needs

What therapies will work for you depends on what troubles you most about your migraines. For most people it is head pain. There are a number of alternative therapies from which to choose, spanning the range from herbs and vitamins to hands-on treatments such as chiropractic therapy, massage, and acupuncture. Then there are those treatments that focus on the mind-body connection, such as biofeedback and meditation, yoga, and tai chi.

As you explore complementary therapies, be certain to discuss your plans and discoveries with your doctor. It is essential that he knows what you are doing.

FIRST PERSON INSIGHTS

Buyer beware

"I have had migraines for 10 years. The medication was okay; the pain only lasted about an hour, but I still got migraines about twice a month and I was getting fed up with them. I was in a health food store and asked the clerk about herbs to help with headaches. She showed me about six different herbs that are supposed to help. Well, I bought them all. I tried them for a while, but they didn't do much. I scheduled massages—that helped with my back, but not my headaches. I even tried hypnosis. I wanted to be in control of my migraines. I finally told my doctor what I was doing. He wasn't happy that I did the herbs on my own without telling him. He said there can be adverse drug interactions. We sat in his office and went through everything. He suggested I stick with vitamins and try biofeedback for the pain."

—Danielle P., Detroit, MI

◆ **Research what's available.** Support groups can be extremely helpful sources of information. Ask the research librarian at your library to help you. Do an Internet search using the name of your illness plus the name of the therapy you want to explore, for example, migraine + biofeedback. (For more information on using the Internet, see Chapter 7).

◆ **Avoid thinking that because something is "natural" it is benign.** Many of the so-called natural or organic substances touted by alterative healers have not been tested, let alone approved, by the FDA. Testimonials and anecdotal evidence do not make something safe. Be especially wary of taking any products or supplements sold directly by a healer. Talk with your doctor before you try anything.

◆ **Stay alert to how you are feeling.** It's tempting to think that you feel lousy all the time. In truth, you have good days and bad days. The more you know about what makes you feel better or worse, the more you can use that knowledge to improve your well-being. Review your health journal (see pages 16–17).

◆ **Bear the expense in mind.** Complementary treatments can cost as much as standard methods—or more, given that many are not covered by insurance plans. Be as frank about your finances as you are about your physical condition. Some practitioners may be willing to negotiate their fees.

◆ **Above all, do not fall for the notion that if the therapy fails, you've failed.** Nothing, not even antibiotics, works equally well for everyone. Give the new therapy a fair trial—some can take a while to show a benefit—but if you are not being helped, give it up and try something else. Or try another person who practices the same therapy; that person may have an insight that makes all the difference.

Herbs and vitamins
nature's medicine chest

There are many herbs and botanicals associated with migraine relief. If you are considering taking any herbal supplement, you should check with your doctor first. There are a number of drug interactions that can occur. Note, too, that herbs and vitamins are not yet regulated by the FDA. That means it is difficult to know the quantity and quality of the supplement you are taking.

One herb study shows that there is a component in an herb called feverfew that actually targets a specific brain chemical involved in the process of inflammation. Other studies have found that feverfew inhibits both the brain chemical serotonin and hormone-like substances known as prostaglandins, both of which are culprits in the migraine process. But feverfew may be involved in rebound headache. And it should never be used if you take a blood thinner, since it may increase bleeding.

Certain vitamins and supplements are showing promising results as well, namely the vitamin riboflavin and the mineral magnesium. Researchers have found that when these two are combined with the herb feverfew, migraines can be prevented in some cases.

Herbal Treatments

If you are interested in considering herbal treatments, talk with your primary care doctor first. Herbs are far from harmless, especially when combined with other over-the-counter and prescription medications.

◆ **Catnip** (*Nepeta cataria*) Cats love this perennial herb that is a member of the mint family. Catnip has been used for centuries to treat respiratory conditions (including coughs, colds, and pneumonia), fever and headaches, and can be valuable in treating sinusitis.

◆ **Chamomile** (*Martricaria chamomilla*) The daisy-like flowers of this annual herb have long been used to treat headaches and calm frazzled nerves, helping relieve tension and TMJ (temporomandibular joint, or jaw joint) headaches. Chamomile is also used against the common cold, insomnia, and indigestion.

◆ **Peppermint** (*Mentha piperita*) Who isn't familiar with this refreshing herb? After all, it's in gum, candy, even toothpaste. But peppermint is more than a tasty flavoring—it has been used for centuries to relieve pain and calm nerves, helping treat tension and TMJ headaches.

◆ **Pleurisy root** (*Asciepis tuberosa*) Although this perennial herb is best known for its ability to treat colds, bronchitis, and of course pleurisy, it is also effective at relieving headaches. Not to be given to children.

◆ **White willow** (*Salix alba*) The bark from this deciduous tree is the origin of our modern-day aspirin. Used for thousands of years to treat pain and fever, willow bark contains salicin, a chemical closely related to the key component of aspirin, salicylic acid. Willow can help relieve various types of headaches. Do not give to children.

Acupuncture
help for head pain

An ancient therapy that arose in China more than 2,000 years ago, acupuncture involves placing fine needles at specific points on the body's surface. According to a 1998 consensus statement from the National Institutes of Health, acupuncture is clearly useful for adults with postoperative and chemotherapy nausea and vomiting, as well as (probably) the nausea of pregnancy. In addition, the National Institutes of Health states that there is promising evidence suggesting the technique can help addiction, stroke rehabilitation, migraine headaches, fibromyalgia, osteoarthritis, low back pain, carpal tunnel syndrome, asthma, and other problems.

A recent study published in the journal Headache found that women who received acupuncture reported fewer migraine attacks during the first four months of treatment, and less need for pain medication during the initial treatment period, than did those who took flunarizine to prevent migraines. However, by the end of six months, there were no differences between the two groups in terms of the number of headaches.

Acupuncture isn't a cure-all. It is best used for people with chronic, long-standing pain problems—such as migraine headaches or musculoskeletal disorders—as well as for those with nonchronic conditions, such as pain related to injuries and other traumas.

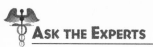

How deep are the needles inserted?

Only a few millimeters. The needles are very fine, and discomfort is minimal.

If I use acupuncture do I need anything else?

Generally, acupuncture is not used as a stand-alone therapy. Practitioners certified in acupuncture may also recommend some herbal treatments, for example.

How do I find a practitioner?

Again, talk to your doctor. Most, but not all, states provide licensing or registration for physician and non-physician acupuncturists. If possible, check to see if your practitioner is certified by the National Certification Commission for Acupuncture and Oriental Medicine. Physicians who use acupuncture in their practices are generally certified by the American Academy of Medical Acupuncture.

Yoga, the "mindful" exercise
using yoga to help you handle your migraines

The goals of yogic exercise are to teach you to stay alert to your body as you exercise and to coordinate your breathing with your movements. For these reasons, many people consider yoga a "mindful" exercise, a form of meditation in motion. But how does that help your migraines? Studies have shown that yoga has a strong antidepressant effect and that it promotes mental and emotional clarity, improves balance, flexibility, strength, and stamina, and relieves chronic muscle aches, eliminates stress, and helps to regulate your metabolism. All exercise helps improve circulation, and that in turn can help stave off some of the complications of migraines. Yoga is especially helpful when used in combination with aerobic exercise, such as brisk walking or bike riding, and traditional strength building, such as working out with light weights.

There are variations in the way yoga is taught. Shop around until you find something that suits you. Some classes are slow paced; others are as lively as a step-aerobics class. Typically, yoga classes can be paid for one at a time, or in sets of five or ten with a discounted price. Some health clubs offer yoga classes, often at no additional cost to the membership price. If you're curious but skeptical, ask to observe a class; you should be able to do this for free. Class lengths vary; a midday class may be 45 minutes, but an evening class may be 60 or 90 minutes long—and priced accordingly.

Qigong and Tai Chi

According to the National Qigong Association, qigong is "an ancient Chinese health care system that integrates physical postures, breathing techniques, and focused intention." Pronounced CHEE gung—and sometimes spelled Chi Kung—the word means "cultivating energy." Tai chi is a form of qigong; both are practiced for health maintenance, healing, and increased vitality. Tai chi is also a martial art, and the sequence of gestures used there help to prepare the person, mentally and physically, for fighting. Both qigong and tai chi consist of a series of dance like gestures that are performed in a specific sequence. The sequence of gestures is called a form, and there are long and short forms of the exercises. In tai chi, the short form takes about ten minutes to complete; it's a bit longer for qigong. Practitioners of the form say that the sense of vitality you feel afterward will last throughout the day.

Chiropractic therapy
spinal adjustments to treat head pain

Chiropractic health care focuses on spinal function and how the spine relates to the nervous system and to overall good health. Despite the fact that some 30 million people seek chiropractic care every year, it still remains a controversial practice in the eyes of some physicians due to chiropractic's nondrug, nonsurgical approach. However, today some physicians are working more closely with doctors of chiropractic, especially when treating back pain.

There is a wealth of evidence that chiropractic adjustments have a significant value in treating back pain. How so? By adjusting the spine and other bones of the body, chiropractors can realign the body to a more natural healthy stance. This can ward off unnecessary muscle strain caused from misaligned bones. Most chiropractors use their hands to make these adjustments. While it is hoped that these subtle adjustments will keep your bones in proper alignment over the long term, they rarely do, and repeat visits are often required.

Some believe that chiropractic therapy can be helpful in treating head pain, especially if the pain is due to problems with muscle tension and misaligned neck vertebrae. So far, studies of its efficacy for head pain vary in their results. However, a report released in 2001 by researchers at the Duke University Evidence-Based Practice Center concluded: "Cervical spine manipulation was associated with significant improvement in headache outcomes in trials involving patients with neck pain and/or neck dysfunction and headache." It should be noted, though, that the study was looking at headaches, not migraine.

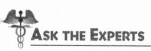

What kind of training do chiropractors receive?

According to the American Chiropractic Association, doctors of chiropractic must complete four to five years at an accredited chiropractic college and pass the national board exam and all exams required by the state in which they practice. They must also meet all individual state licensing requirements in order to become doctors of chiropractic.

How do I find a chiropractor?

Finding a chiropractor may be as simple as asking your medical doctor for a referral. Otherwise, the American Chiropractic Association has a doctor finder on its Web site at **www.acatoday.org**.

I think my health insurance covers visits to a chiropractor. How do I know for sure?

Very simply call your health insurer and find out what it covers. Some insurers do cover chiropractic visits but cap the number of visits.

Massage and bodywork
the lowdown on getting a rubdown

Bodywork is the catchall word for a range of physical therapies that involve manipulation of the body. As with other complementary therapies, bodywork is very helpful at relieving symptoms, especially any stress-related symptoms. Stress does take a physical toll on our bodies.

People who practice therapeutic massage generally avoid the words "masseuse" and "masseur" and instead call themselves massage therapists. Their ads will state that they practice therapeutic, medical, or sports massage, and in states where the practice is regulated by the government, the abbreviation LMT (licensed massage therapist) may follow the person's name. Another string of letters to look for is NCTMB. This means that the therapist has received at least 500 hours of training and has passed a qualifying exam administered by the National Certification Board for Therapeutic Massage and Bodywork. In states where massage is a licensed health practice, your insurance company may reimburse some of the costs.

In general, massage means Swedish massage and/or Shiatsu (see page 161), and bodywork encompasses a wide range of other physically based therapies. Another distinction, albeit a fine one, is that massage is often limited to physical manipulation, and bodywork is based on the idea that the body is composed of energy fields and channels and that blocked energy causes or exacerbates disease.

The different practices vary in intensity and therapeutic benefits; almost all of them can be successfully administered while you are clothed. Also, different therapists have different "touches"—some work gently, others work vigorously. Never hire someone to hurt you. Ask the therapist how much discomfort you might experience as an inherent part of the treatment, and if the therapist is working too deeply, speak up.

Here's a look at some popular bodywork therapies. To get more information or for help in locating a practitioner, see Helpful resources (page 162).

Swedish massage Originally intended to help improve blood circulation and encourage drainage of the lymph system, this technique uses gliding, kneading, tapping, or vibrating strokes for gentle or penetrating muscle massage. It is especially helpful for tension relief and relaxation.

Myofascial therapy This is a general term for a number of techniques that manipulate soft tissue—muscle fibers (myo-) and fascia, the connective tissue that holds muscle fibers in place—to relieve trigger points, localized areas that are painful themselves or provoke pain in other areas.

Rolfing Developed by Ida P. Rolf, a biochemist, who called the process Structural Integration, it is a form of deep manipulation of the body's soft tissues to balance energy and relieve chronic pain and stress. Practitioners are trained and certified by the Rolf Institute in Colorado.

Shiatsu (acupressure) A component of traditional Chinese medicine. Practitioners use fingertip pressure on specific points along the body's energy channels to release blocks, restore balance, and encourage health.

CranioSacral therapy (CST) Developed by an osteopath, Dr. John E. Upledger. Practitioners gently manipulate the skull, the sacrum, and the nerve endings in the scalp. It is helpful for back and neck pain, headache, sinus infections, stress and tension, chronic fatigue, and fibromyalgia. Practitioners are trained and certified by the Upledger Institute in Florida.

The Trager Approach Non-intrusive massage and movement reeducation, focusing on integrating the mind and body to relieve anxiety. Practitioners are trained and certified by the Trager Institute in Ohio.

Helpful resources

Beyond the Relaxation Response
by Herbert Benson, M.D.

Full Catastrophe Living
by Jon Kabat-Zinn

What Your Doctor May Not Tell You about Migraines
by Alexander Mauskop, M.D. and Barry Fox Ph.D.

National Center for Complementary and Alternative Medicine (NCCAM)
National Institutes of Health
Bethesda, MD 20892
Tel: 888 644-7227
www.nccam.nih.gov
This government agency provides information about and sponsors research in complementary therapies.

American Council on Science and Health
1995 Broadway, Second floor
New York, NY 10023-5860
Tel: 212 362-7044
Fax: 212 362-4919
www.acsh.org

www.alternativehealing.org
This site is full of advice and explanations about every kind of alternative treatment under the sun.

American College for the Advancement of Medicine
Tel: 714 583-7666
This organization is an excellent resource for finding alternative, licensed doctors practicing in your area.

www.holisticonline.com

Cutting-edge Research

Improved triptans
new drugs are working wonders

The problem with today's standard migraine drugs, known as triptans, is not their effectiveness, but their side effects. In one study, nearly 1,200 people who got migraines were questioned about the medications they took. Of those taking triptans, patients listed as common side effects sleepiness and fatigue, racing heartbeat, nausea, and difficulty in thinking. In short, the cure is often worse than the disease. The other problem with triptans is that they are not advisable (what doctors call contraindicated) for people who have heart disease and/or risk factors for stroke. Unfortunately, these are very common, which means that a lot of people who get migraines are not allowed to take triptans to prevent a migraine. If you have heart disease or are at risk for stroke, triptans aren't for you.

The solution is simple: Come up with a triptan drug that has fewer side effects. Here's where research comes in, particularly research that is focused on small proteins called receptors that are found on the surface of cells. Receptors play an important role in the ability of our cells to talk to each other. For example, if nerve cell A wants nerve cell B to do something, nerve cell A releases a chemical messenger that travels to a receptor located on nerve cell B. That receptor will then activate the nerve cell. It's a lock-and-key dynamic.

One chemical used by nerve cells to transmit information is called serotonin. Serotonin is present throughout the body, as are serotonin receptors known as 5-hydroxytriptamine (5-HT) receptors. What interests researchers are the serotonin receptors that are found on the terminals of the trigeminal nerve—a large nerve that supplies sensation to much of the face and head, including the eye and the lower and upper jaw. During the migraine process, certain brain structures are activated that, in turn, release several chemicals. One of these chemicals is called CGRP (calictonin gene related peptide). CGRP activates receptors on blood vessel walls in the brain and on the trigeminal nerve terminals. A blood vessel dilates. The trigeminal nerve activates. The result? Pain.

Enter the triptans. These drugs have the ability to link to the trigeminal nerve terminals and block the release of CGRP. Triptans also link to receptors on the blood vessel walls. Essentially, triptans have the ability to reduce blood vessel inflammation and trigeminal nerve activation. The result? No pain. The problem with older triptan drugs, such as sumatriptan, is that they link up to a number of different receptors, serotonin included. They are nonselective. The result is an array of side effects, such as chest pain, cough, fever, sneezing, sore throat, a feeling of heaviness in the chest, irregular heartbeat. And the list goes on.

The goal of drug research is to achieve greater selectivity in the blocked receptors. Today, there are a host of triptans available. The triptans are generally similar in efficacy—providing relief to about two-thirds of migraine sufferers who take the drugs. Some seem to work better for the menstrual migraine (see Chapter 4); others have a seemingly longer duration and quicker onset. But, like the painkillers before them, the triptans deliver their best results when taken early in an attack.

What's behind the aura?

Just recently, researchers demonstrated the firing of the nerve cells by introducing a low-intensity magnetic field into the brain, through the back of the head, causing the cells to fire off in people prone to migraines. What those migraine patients saw were bright flashing lights signaling the beginning of the migraine aura.

What causes the excitability of the cells that leads to migraine? Some researchers speculate that it may be due to low magnesium levels in the brain, or even to nerve cells that require only low energy levels to set them off. To offset the deficiency, some doctors are prescribing magnesium to their patients. Researchers have had some luck with vitamins like thiamine and riboflavin, which, for some people who get migraines, seem to decrease the number of episodes.

Old drugs, new uses
using antiepilepsy drugs to ward off migraines

One of the most exciting approaches in the search for ways to prevent migraines has been the study of epilepsy drugs. They seem to calm the highly excitable brain nerve cells of people who get migraines.

Divalproex is an anticonvulsant drug often used for migraine prevention for those who do not respond to other treatments. But a new drug may prove more effective. In a study of more than 400 migraine sufferers given varying doses of the anticonvulsant drug topiramate or a placebo for four months, about half found their number and duration of migraines cut in half. The drug—unlike other anticonvulsants or mood stabilizers—also had the unexpected side benefit of decreased appetite and weight loss.

Though patients with epilepsy must take the medication for the duration of their illness, some people who get migraines may experience longer-term relief from short-term use of the drug. Early research is showing that the drug may "turn off" the migraine process in some patients after a drug regimen of three to six months. Topiramate isn't without side effects, though researchers are finding that the side effects—including anxiety, a feeling of pins and needles, and even language problems—are dose dependent and temporary, or disappear once medication is discontinued.

New Avenues of Attack

The discovery that migraines are caused not by abnormal blood vessels but by a unique electrical disorder of brain cells, means researchers have many new avenues to explore. For example, researchers are looking at the possibility of reducing levels of glutamate—a brain chemical that activates nerve cells—which means it has receptors. So one potential avenue of exploration is choosing or targeting a specific glutamate receptor with a medication. Because blocking a glutamate receptor would not affect blood vessels, there would be no blood vessel constriction or possible vascular side effects. If a drug is developed in the future, it may have the distinct advantage of being available to more people who get migraines.

Other researchers are looking at targeting nitric oxide (NO) a small molecule that helps in the control of blood vessel dilation and constriction. Some studies show that the heart pill nitroglycerin, which opens constricted blood vessels by releasing NO, causes migraine episodes in many people who get migraines. So some researchers are looking at ways to block NO from forming. Others are looking at ways to stop the electrical activity that spreads throughout the brain at the beginning of a migraine attack.

Many of these studies are in the very earliest of stages. But as science learns more about the migraine, it's inevitable that new drugs will be developed from these and other studies.

Botox for migraines
get rid of a wrinkle and stop a migraine

Science and serendipity seem to have a lot in common. Take a look at injectable botulism toxin, better known as Botox, which is used to paralyze facial muscles and in the process ease wrinkles. The link between Botox and migraines was first discovered when a plastic surgeon found that patients he injected with the toxin to help get rid of wrinkles received an unexpected side effect: no more headaches.

Now research teams across the country are studying the effects of Botox on people who get migraines. And the news is pretty good, though scientists are the first to admit they don't know exactly why Botox seems to work. Initially, doctors thought its effect on headaches was simply a result of relaxing tense muscles in the head and neck. Indeed, that may play a role in why Botox works for some patients, but it's really secondary, since muscle tension isn't the cause of a headache.

Botox was approved by the FDA in the late 1980s for treatment of eye muscle disorders. More recently, Botox was approved for reducing the severity of glabeller lines, or frown lines, on the face. Though doctors are still trying to figure out the optimal dose of the toxin for migraine treatment, many neurologists, dermatologists, and others are using the drug off label for migraine, meaning that until the FDA grants approval for the drug, it is not covered by medical insurance.

Some of the study results are intriguing. In one study, patients who had already tried up to three medicines for their headaches, with little effect, were given one to four Botox treatments spaced at three-month intervals. Among those patients who received four treatments, 92 percent reported an improvement; 84 percent of the patients reported improvement if they received fewer treatments.

Though early results of clinical trials are encouraging, there needs to be more research before Botox will be considered a primary treatment for migraine and other forms of headache. Right now, for example, doctors don't know who will respond to Botox and who won't respond. Plus, Botox is very expensive. Treatments can run anywhere from $500 to $900 every three months. And you probably won't get any help from your insurer, since Botox is not approved for use in migraine. However, do check with your insurer in any case. There are some patients who have gotten some coverage, especially those who have another condition, such as muscle spasms of the eye, for which Botox is already approved.

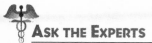

ASK THE EXPERTS

I'd like to try Botox for my migraines. How do I go about getting it?

For cosmetic reasons, you can see a plastic surgeon or a dermatologist. When it comes to migraines, remember, Botox is still being researched. Talk to your doctor, and perhaps she will make a referral so you can see if Botox helps you. You can also check to see if there is an ongoing clinical trial in your region. Perhaps you can be a study participant.

I've heard about migraine surgery. Is there anything to that?

Some researchers are studying the feasibility of removing the bulk of the muscles called the corrugator supercilii, that are underneath the eyebrows, in patients whose migraines were eliminated by Botox for a specific period of time. In one small study, 95 percent of 24 patients reported an improvement in their migraines: 46 percent reported complete elimination of the migraine, and at least 50 percent reported an improvement in the severity and frequency of migraines. This all came about because patients who have facelifts sometimes have an added benefit: a reduction in the frequency of migraines. Much larger patient populations need to be studied before migraine surgery becomes migraine gospel.

Joining a clinical trial
clinical trials offer a chance to make a difference

Getting a drug from the petri dish to the medicine chest would not happen if it weren't for the thousands of people who become study participants in the clinical trial. It's through the clinical trial that researchers are able to determine which medications work and which don't.

How exactly do clinical trials work? Let's say a drug company develops a brand new compound. First it must be tested for safety. The new drug will be tested on non-human subjects. If the drug does not pass muster, further testing doesn't happen. The drug is scrapped, and it's back to the drawing board. But if the drug has no adverse effects, the next step will be small trials with human subjects. The drug company will file an application with the Food and Drug Administration (FDA), and an independent review board will play watchdog, ensuring that all study subjects are protected. That means that the drug company must adequately explain the purpose of the trial, and the benefits and risks, and that informed consent has been given by all study participants.

This is the earliest phase of drug study, and it's called a Phase I study. The purpose of the Phase I study is to gather safety information as well as any other pertinent data, such as side effects. Clinical trials progress through different stages. In simplest terms, a Phase I trial, for example, studies the safety of a specific new treatment, and identifies any side effects. These trials are very small, and participation is limited. If all goes well, a drug will move into Phase II. During this phase, all the work from Phase I continues, but larger groups of patients are then studied. The next stage is called Phase III, and thousands of people participate. The goal is to figure out how well a new drug compares to older treatments.

In Phase III, scientists look closely at the drug's effectiveness in large populations of people who get migraines. The researchers will look for side effects, optimal dosing, and of course, effectiveness. In later stages of the trial, the drug may even be compared to a similar agent already on the market. All this testing takes time. Some estimates show that it may take as long as 14 years to get a new drug approved.

To find out about clinical trials for migraine, ask your doctor, especially if you are not responding to current treatment. Another good resource is the Internet. Go online to **www.migraine-clinical-trials.com**. Just be aware that the team in charge of a specific study will have very specific parameters regarding potential study participants. Not every patient with migraine will meet all the parameters for every migraine study.

FIRST PERSON INSIGHTS

I was desperate

"I was one of the first people to take part in a clinical trial of sumatriptan. My doctor told me about the trial since he was one of the doctors trying to determine whether this new class of drugs was worth anything. I was really desperate to do something. I wasn't thinking about advancing medicine or some drug company's agenda. I just wanted to try something new, something that might actually help me with the pain. I admit the trial was kind of grueling. There was a lot of paperwork. A lot of visits back to the doctor. A lot of work on my part. I thought I'd just have to pop a pill. The trial lasted about six months. And there was no pill. I had to inject the drug. I don't know if I helped other people or not. All I know is that I helped myself. And I think that's okay, too."

—Donna J., Nashville, TN

Helpful resources

Migraine: A Neuroinflammatory Disease? (Progress in Inflammation Research)
by Egiluis L. H. Spierings

Reducing the Burden of Headache (Frontiers in Headache Research)
by Jes Olesen

Here are some of the best sites to keep bookmarked:
www.migraine-clinical-trials.com

www.centerwatch.com/patient/ studies/cat100.html

www.veritasmedicine.com

www.clinicaltrials.gov

Stress and the Migraine

What is stress?
it's not just a built-in survival mechanism

Stress has become the watchword for a number of medical problems today. It seems that stress can cause certain illnesses as well as worsen your symptoms once you become ill. How does that happen? The answer lies in the complex nature of stress, or rather our complex reaction to it. While scientists have learned a great deal more about the nature of stress in the past few years, they are still baffled by it. One of the most puzzling aspects of stress is that its effect on our bodies is based on how we perceive stressful situations. Some stressors can help us perform at our peak abilities; other stressors can be debilitating. It's all in the eye of the beholder. So far the one thing researchers agree upon is that the number one reason for negative stress is the perception of not being in control. Not having control over one's life or environment can be a very threatening feeling and can easily trigger the stress response. What scientists have now discovered is that the feeling of powerlessness can be both short and long term.

A perceived short-term threat

This stressor could be a lunging tiger, an oncoming car, or an angry boss. Reacting to threats is so critical to our survival that our bodies are designed to either fight or flee the threat. Here's how how our bodies handle it. When a threat is perceived, the brain's hypothalamus sends out an alarm to the sympathetic nervous system to release adrenaline into the blood stream. This increases your heart rate and blood pressure so you can run or fight. It also drains blood from the brain. That means the brain is getting less oxygen, which in turn makes rational thinking a lot harder. (Ever wonder why people sometimes freeze in the face of danger or do something really irrational? It's because they get so light-headed they literally cannot think of what to do.) Note: The perceived threat is always in the eye of the beholder. The stress response will occur whether the threat is real or imagined. (This is why your heart races during a scary movie.)

The brain also signals the adrenal glands to release epinephrine and nor-epinephrine hormones. These hormones increase the glucose levels in the blood so that muscles can effectively respond. This is why some people can perform incredible feats of strength in a crisis.

Once the threat has passed, the brain issues an all-clear signal. Neurons, special cells in the brain, send out signals to the major organs to return to normal. This allows the digestive system to go back to the business of digesting food, and the heart's rate and blood pressure to return to a calmer beat. Essentially, the body is told to relax—the threat has passed. If the threat lasted for a few minutes, ideally it will take just a few minutes to return to normal.

Women and Stress

Women react differently than men
For the past fifty years, stress research was done on male animals. It was from their response to various stressors that researchers came up with the catch phrase "fight or flight." That changed in 1998 when researcher Shelley E. Taylor thought to study the stress response in female animals. Dr. Taylor found that females responded differently to nonlife-threatening stress, particularly if they were tending young off-spring. The female animals did not become nearly as alarmed as their male counterparts. In fact, their reaction was to tend to their young and to seek comfort in other females. Dr. Taylor went on to test her theory on men and women and found that in general men tend to isolate themselves when they feel stressed, while women confide their problems to each other. As Dr. Taylor describes it in her book, *The Tending Instinct*, women "tend and befriend."

Chronic stress
be alert to coping patterns

What happens when a perceived threat lingers for days or weeks? Long-term negative stressors, such as going through a messy divorce, becoming ill, or getting laid off from work, go on for months. This means the all-clear signal is never given by the brain, so the body never gets a chance to return to equilibrium. It's as if the body is on a constant state of alert. Over time, this can take a physical toll on the body, especially if these stressors are perceived to be negative threats. A kind of learned helplessness can set in, a feeling that events are out of one's control, which can lead to lowered motivation, self-esteem, and initiative. Again, perception is key. This is why some people thrive on such stressors as deadlines for a project they are passionate about, while others who don't feel emotionally involved or in control of their work feel stressed out.

When it comes to long-term stress, having a sense of control is key. Long-term negative stress can lead to bouts of anxiety, aggression, and depression. Some scientists believe that chronic stress has a harmful effect on the immune system and the endocrine system, making people more vulnerable to illness and infection. Whether you have an illness or not, when it comes to chronic stress you need to work on improving your coping skills.

So, how do you cope with long-term stress? For starters, look at how you have coped in the past with other chronic stressors, especially negative ones. Did you isolate yourself from friends and family? Did you seek out comfort foods? Sleep a lot? Fall into bad habits, such as overeating or drinking? Try and see if there is a pattern to how you coped. It's also a good idea to recall how your parents or other significant caregivers handled negative stressors. You may have internalized their coping responses and not realized it.

Negative Coping Responses

There are several negative coping responses that we all have used at one time or another when dealing with long-term stress. Here is a roundup:

- ◆ **Deny your problems**. This is a common response for many people—they simply ignore their problems. Often, to help take their minds off their problems, they throw themselves into their work or social life.

- ◆ **Dwell on your problems**. Again, this is usually a learned response. Did your parents or caregivers fret excessively over your health as you were growing up? Or did they ignore your health completely? If they sought either of these extremes, you may find yourself obsessing about your health. If these thoughts become chronic, you should see a therapist who can help you break the pattern of obsessive rumination.

- ◆ **Procrastinate in decision-making**. Instead of thinking through the problems at hand, you endlessly analyze the situations, and talk about the same problems and solutions over and over again with friends and family.

- ◆ **Seek thrills**. Here you look for thrills or experiences to distract you from your problems.

- ◆ **Get angry and lash out at others**. This is known as displaced aggression. It's where you take out your anger at being ill on others and over-react to their responses.

- ◆ **Withdraw**. This can take the form of physically or emotionally withdrawing from others. Often people under chronic stress will cope by sleeping excessively or simply by disengaging from the world.

- ◆ **Overindulge**. Food is used as a drug to mask fears as well as boredom. Too much alcohol is another way to cope with all the problems of chronic stress, and so is smoking too many cigarettes or cigars.

Assault on mind and body
stress can lead to other physical ailments

The event that triggers stress can be good (a promotion) or bad (a diagnosis of a chronic illness). Hundreds of studies show that stress aggravates illness, chronic or episodic, life-threatening or curable. Uncontrolled stress can weaken the immune system and make a person more prone to other health problems, such as colds, flu, general malaise, and fatigue.

◆ Chronic stress can exacerbate or even trigger hair loss, make wounds heal more slowly, and cause a person to become prone to adult acne, rashes, eczema, hives, and other dermatological problems.

◆ High stress can lead to binge eating, resulting in obesity, which can lead to a host of problems, such as heart disease and diabetes, among others.

◆ High stress levels—along with negative emotions—release high levels of cortisol and homocysteine (a by-product of protein metabolism linked to heart disease). Blood pressure and cholesterol levels go up.

◆ Reproduction can be difficult since chronic stress compromises the reproductive hormones for both men and women.

◆ Severe gastrointestinal problems are also common, from exacerbation of the symptoms of ulcers to aggravation of already sensitive bowels.

◆ Chronic muscle tension due to chronic stress can make arthritis flare-ups worse and exacerbate lower back problems.

◆ The chronically stressed can have mild memory loss and problems with concentrating or organizing thoughts.

◆ If you have some bad habits, they will get worse with chronic stress. Smoking, binge drinking, and drug abuse have all been linked to chronic stress.

Stress as a Migraine Trigger

Though migraine is not a stress-related illness, stress can be a migraine trigger, like caffeine, chocolate, an errant wind, even a change in temperature. So, for that matter, can lack of stress—when you're on vacation, for example, and have changed your sleep habits. You're supposed to be relaxing, but you get a migraine. It seems that people who get migraines just can't win.

Many successful business people, politicians, medical professionals, and other high achievers have migraines. If they couldn't handle stress, they wouldn't be good at their jobs. On the other hand, some of the stresses of a high-pressure job—lack of sleep and poor eating habits due to overwork among others—can trigger an episode.

Smart coping strategies
find positive ways to cope with chronic problems

Having a chronic illness can tap your coping reserves. Your old favorite coping standbys may work, but not for long. The challenge of coping with a long-term illness is understanding how to live with it. This calls for a new way of looking at your health and at illness. Since there is no cure yet for many chronic illnesses, the goal becomes the reduction of discomfort. That means really listening to your symptoms and addressing them. Your goal is simply to improve your quality of life. Here are some coping tips to help you on your way:

Create a migraine retreat. We all need a place of our own to retreat to when the going gets tough. This is especially vital when you have a migraine. For most of us, this is our bedroom. When a migraine strikes, you need to be able to convert your bedroom into a soundproof, darkened room (get heavy drapes).

Get organized. Time management becomes a tool you can use when you have a chronic illness. Your time and energy are now precious commodities that should not be wasted. Learn how to separate those things you really need to do from those you can spread out over time or delegate to others.

Develop healthy habits. Ironically, people often become healthier once health problems have been diagnosed. This may be because they suddenly stop taking their health for granted and turn negative habits into healthy ones, such as eating healthy (see pages 136-139) or quitting smoking.

Make attitude adjustments. Life with any chronic problem can make the world a dour place. Put some humor back in your life. Rent funny movies, or read humorous books and magazines.

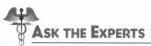

I have to travel for work. How can I cut down on stress while I am on the road?

Traveling is a big stressor, and doubly so if you have to manage a chronic illness while you are on the road. It's smart to be proactive and plan ahead as much as possible. For starters, create a mini-health file with the phone numbers and contact information for all of the people on your support team (see Chapter 6). Make sure to bring extra medication just in case. Next, don't just pack for your trip. Bring a bit of home with you. Include a pair of comfortable jeans or a favorite shawl. Some people who hate to travel bring photos of their family and put them in their hotel room. Don't forget to bring a novel, computer games, knitting, or whatever you like to do to relax. Your goal is to detoxify the stress of travel with things that instantly signal comfort and relaxation.

Also, as a person with migraine, the most important thing you can do is to try and keep your routines the same. That means to try to keep the same sleep-wake schedule as you do at home. Try to eat meals at the same time. And try to avoid those specific triggers that may jumpstart a migraine.

Take a stress inventory
how are migraine stressors affecting you?

No one wants to think that his or her stress levels are out of control, but sometimes it is necessary to confront the stress of a health problem head-on. One way is to take a personal stress inventory by asking some tough questions, especially if you feel your migraine is overwhelming your life—despite treatment. Consider the following questions as they may apply to you.

- Are you having difficulty accepting a diagnosis of migraine and the fact that there is no cure?

- Are you getting disgusted with trying new medications, none of which seem to work for you?

- Are you spending a lot of time—to the exclusion of all else—researching migraine and other illnesses?

- If your migraine is responding to treatment, do you hesitate to plan social outings with friends or family because you're afraid of another episode?

These questions aren't scientific. But they do provide a starting point to assess how the stressors of living with a migraine may be affecting you. Again, it doesn't really matter if your migraine is once a month, three times a week, an hour filled with pain, or days. The point is that you have an extra stress in your life—migraine. If any of these questions seem particularly pertinent to you, talk to your health professional. She may be able to allay some of your fears. A support group (see page 106 and 190) can also be helpful in allowing you to share your experiences with others who get migraines. And if no one close to you understands the disease, educate them. (See page 188.) Stress is part of life. Do not let the stress of the migraine take control of your life.

Sharing Your Health News

Don't be surprised if when you mention that you get migraines your listener immediately cuts you off and tells you about her friend's experience with migraines. Why does that happen, you wonder? Your friend may be trying to gain a sense of involvement in your plight and show that she has some experience with or knowledge of your situation. But it can also be a way to create distance between you and her. By telling another person's story, she takes you out of the spotlight and puts her friend in it. This can give her a needed sense of control and distance while she absorbs your news. Ideally, you want a friend to be a good listener—maybe ask a few questions but still keep the focus on you. Since it can be uncomfortable to hear about a total stranger's problems when you have just revealed your own, tell your friend you are not ready to talk about your illness in such detail, and simply change the subject. Be sure to tell your friend that you would appreciate that she not share your news with others, if that is what you wish.

Learning to relax
beat chronic stress at its own game

Our bodies are brilliantly designed to handle stress. They are also designed to handle relaxation. In fact, both the stress response and the relaxation response are hardwired into our brains. Doctors are just now beginning to understand the power of relaxation upon the body—both to rejuvenate and to heal.

Think back to a time when you felt truly relaxed. What was going on? You were probably in a quiet, comfortable space where you had no pressures to do anything and could sit back and enjoy the day. You felt peaceful and at one with the world. For most people that is the definition of a vacation. Here's the news flash: To be healthy, your body needs a little vacation every day. How do you achieve that? Here are some tips:

Quiet time Carve out ten minutes of the day to simply sit quietly and be. Meditation practices are very helpful in teaching people how to quiet their minds and relax. See pages 146–147 for more on this.

Deep breathing When we are stressed, our breathing becomes shortened, so much so that we can hyperventilate when faced with acute stress. Counter this natural instinct by purposefully taking four deep breaths every time you feel stressed. Breathe in through your nose, hold the breath for five seconds, and then release the air through your mouth.

Exercise Chronic muscle tension is part and parcel of a chronic stress response. Counteract it by taking a walk or playing a round of tennis. Your goal is to keep your body limber and to keep it moving. For a more relaxing exercise, consider taking a class in yoga or tai chi (see pages 156–157 for more information). Note: Massage is a great way to help rid your muscles of stress-related tension. (See pages 160–161.)

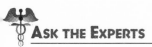

Ask the Experts

I have been anxious for so long, I don't think anything will help. What can I do?

If you have been enduring chronic stressors for a long period of time, trying to relax overnight is not going to work. In fact, it will just make you more stressed. You need to retrain your body to feel and behave relaxed. Consider taking a short-term workshop to help you learn to how to relax. Your doctor can refer you to a stress clinic or a stress specialist. You can take courses on stress management. The American Management Association offers two-day workshops on managing stress; call them at 800 262-9699. Or try your local YMCA or YMHA; they usually offer stress management classes.

I hear writing about stressful events helps you get over them. True?

Some studies show that writing about stressful issues or traumatic experiences can help improve the immune system. Use your health journal (see pages 16–17) to write about your concerns.

Getting People to Understand

It can be hard to try to explain what it's like to have a chronic health problem to those who have never had one, especially one like migraines where you don't look sick. Try to find an analogy that works. Most working people can relate to the experience of being laid off. Having a chronic illness is a lot like getting laid off. In both cases, it happens through no fault of your own. And there is a sense of being an outsider—you miss your work routine and feel cut off from the "normal" working world. You also are concerned about your future and are anxious to get back to work.

Your partner's concerns
how chronic illness can impact relationships

When one-half of a couple has a chronic illness, both members usually need to reassess their partnership. If it's a temporary illness, then it's usually a question of juggling practical matters, such as who will pick up the kids while you're at the doctor. But when symptoms are no longer signs of a temporary illness, but the manifestation of a lingering health problem, a bigger reassessment is needed. When it comes to handling the ordeals of migraine, couples need to look at each partner's role and responsibilities in the relationship. You need to state what changes need to be made. This may mean reassigning roles, be it cleaning duties or paying the bills, when a migraine strikes. Often couples fall into the trap where one becomes the dominant caregiver and the other becomes the professional patient. Try to avoid that dynamic because it usually leads to resentment on both sides. It's a good idea to have your spouse come along with you on a doctor's visit so that he or she sees firsthand what it is like to be a patient.

Money may become an issue if you do not have adequate health insurance or need to cut back on work. Sometimes migraines can affect your love life, because they can typically strike following sex. Talk about your concerns and listen to your partner. The important thing is to keep the lines of communication open and not to shut down. A good therapist, knowledgeable about the effects of chronic disease on sexuality, may be able to help you work through these issues. To find a therapist for your particular concern, start at the American Association of Sex Educators, Counselors, and Therapists (**www.aasect.org**).

◆ **Know Your Migraine:** Some studies show that those patients who are most successful in dealing with a chronic illness are those who learn about their conditions. Though the Internet can be fraught with misinformation (see Chapter 7), more than half of patients with chronic illness use the Internet as a source of information, and most find it helpful. Nearly 90 percent, however, say their doctors are the most help, especially if they take the time to explain the illness and what to expect in the future.

◆ **Be Aware of Depression:** If you are feeling helpless and hopeless, that depressive state can be a real barrier to success. People with chronic illnesses have a 25 to 33 percent chance of suffering from depression in addition to their other condition(s); this is a significantly higher risk than found in the general population. Those people who get migraines seem to have higher rates of depression, and conversely, depressed patients seem to have more migraines. Researchers aren't quite sure of the correlation, but one thing is clear: Depression is a problem that needs to be treated. Patients and their caregivers need to be educated about the signs and symptoms of depression and to alert the physician when problems arise. Physicians, in turn, need to be on the lookout for signs of depression.

◆ **Get Off the Couch:** Taking some form of action immediately after a diagnosis seems to provide the best long-term results for living well. People who have successfully managed their chronic condition responded to their diagnosis by thinking about lifestyle changes that may be necessary and how to adapt to those changes. Those who were less successful tended to avoid the issue, deny the diagnosis, or just withdraw, wishing their condition would just go away.

Is all stress bad? There is something called positive stress, or eustress. Positive stress provides extra energy to get a job done, for example, since it boosts productivity. Actually, a low level of stress may be what induced you to take your migraine more seriously, forcing you to find out more about your illness, to see a medical professional, and to develop a plan for today and the future.

Talking about it
learn how to talk about your needs

For a lot of people, talking about their health issues is torturous. They just don't know how to do it. They don't want to come across as whiners, nor do they want to seem overly dramatic. And so they say nothing. If this sounds familiar, then it's time to learn how to talk about having a chronic illness like the migraine. If you have frequent migraines that are very severe, for example, you should tell your friends and family about what you have learned about the disease. Even if you have mild and infrequent migraines, you still have a chronic illness. Plus, even the mildest form of the disease can be triggered by something as innocuous as a piece of chocolate or a glass of wine. Chances are your friends, family members, and colleagues will probably ask you why you don't want to try that scrumptious chocolate cake or a glass of wine. So a chronic illness, even one like the migraine, should be talked about. Here are a few tips to make it easier:

1. Pick the time and place to talk. You need to set a time and place that is comfortable for you. Don't get backed into talking about your illness when you are not ready. You need to feel in control of the conversation; picking the place and time will help you feel in charge.

2. Rehearse out loud in front of a mirror before you actually talk to your spouse or friends. Simply saying the words ahead of time can help you get over your shyness.

3. Set the terms and limits of the information you want to share. You are the one in charge here; don't let anyone take over the conversation and ask you invasive questions. Simply call a halt to the questions and say you don't feel comfortable answering them right now. Also, set the terms of your information. If you don't want this information shared with others, then say so.

Learn how to not talk about it.

It's only natural to assume that because something interests you intensely, then it must also interest everyone else. And if that something is as all-important as your migraine, your family and close friends will surely want to know every detail, and even casual acquaintances will be fascinated by the dramatic story line. Wrong. Remind yourself every day that a good conversationalist is first of all a good listener. Ask questions about things that interest other people, and listen—really listen—to the answers. Have things to talk about besides you and your health concerns.

Five Rules for Talking About Your Illness

1. "How are you?" is a greeting, not a request for medical news. Just because you have a chronic illness, there is no reason to change your usual response. Wait until someone asks specifically about your illness before telling them about it.

2. Fit the answer to your audience. Have a short version and a long version ready. Your spouse may want to hear every detail the minute you come from your doctor's visit. But your colleagues want only a summary version.

3. Watch for eyes glazing over. Someone has asked about your illness and seems really interested. So you launch into the long version. Watch for signs of boredom. Does she fidget? Glance around? If you pause or ask a question, is there a slight delay before you have her attention again?

4. After three minutes, change the subject. Even the most loving friend may not be able to take in every detail of an extended medical report. Give her a break. If someone is really interested, she'll return to the subject.

5. Use humor. Have a couple of jokes handy to break up your monologue, or provide an exit line.

Find a support group
but first, decide what you want

Millions of people, sooner or later, echo the catchy Beatles refrain, "Help. I need somebody." Indeed, some 25 million people will participate in self-help groups at some time during the course of their lives, according to one study. With the Internet and online support groups, that number is expected to rise, as a growing network of support becomes available for the masses of individuals who find in-person groups physically problematic or emotionally uncomfortable. Today, about three to four percent of the U.S. population, or between 8 and 11 million people, participate in self-help groups each year.

When you're facing a tough challenge—coping with an illness, caring for a family member, grieving over the death of a loved one—you need all the help you can get. One of the places you can turn to is a support group, online or up close and personal at a local community center or hospital.

Things to keep in mind when looking for a support group:

◆ Figure out what you want. Are you looking for more facts, emotional support, or a combination of both? Every support group, depending on its moderator (both on- and off-line) and participants, will have a slightly different flavor. Some may be focused on research, if that is what participants want. Others will be solely for emotional support.

◆ Make sure the group is reputable, either conducted by a local hospital or sponsored by a medical professional. Online support groups generally have moderators, who may or may not be migraine sufferers themselves, and such groups are often visited by medical professionals. Most of the good sites have rules about spamming participants with unproven remedies, or hawking other miracle cures. Message boards are a great resource, but remember to take everything you hear with a grain of salt when it comes to medical advice. You don't know who is on the other side of the Send button.

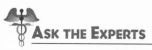

ASK THE EXPERTS

Can pets reduce stress?

There is some evidence that pets can reduce stress and hypertension. In one six-month study at the State University of New York at Buffalo SUNY Buffalo, participants who adopted a dog or cat saw blood pressure caused by mental stress rise less than those who did not have a pet. Both the group with pets and the one without took an ACE Inhibitor, a commonly prescribed means of controlling overall blood pressure. But when asked to take stress-inducing tests, such as giving a speech or doing arithmetic problems, the pet-owning group fared better when their blood pressure was taken.

Why do people always tell me to breathe deeply whenever I get stressed or upset or angry?

When you get upset, it is usually because something did not go your way or something happened that was out of your control. Either way, the main problem is that you are out of control. One way to counteract that feeling of powerlessness is to do something that you can control, namely your breathing. By concentrating on your breath and breathing in deeply and exhaling slowly, you are not only getting more oxygen into your blood, but also telling yourself that, despite all else, you are in control.

Migraine and the job
providing proper medical care is smart business

Lisa M. has a migraine. She's weak from vomiting; she's lying on her bed in the dark waiting for the medicine to ease the throbbing pressure in her head. Even though she's taking a drug that works for her (the most effective available), she's wiped out. It will be a day before she can go to work. She called in sick, the second time in two months. The sixth time this year. Lisa believes her coworkers are angry. Worse yet, she thinks her boss is ready to let her go.

Sound familiar? If you're a person who gets severe migraines, one of the toughest stressors is the job. Migraine is a major cause of lost productivity, totaling nearly $6 billion in missed work and physician visits and more than 157 million lost workdays a year. In a study of some 135,000 people who get migraines, about 11 percent were bedridden an average of 1.6 days, and 9 percent were restricted from normal activities for an average of 2.4 days per two-week period of observation. An 18-month study in a managed-care setting found people with migraines generating nearly twice as many medical claims and 2.5 times more prescription claims than those without migraine.

Having an understanding boss and coworkers certainly helps. Some companies are increasingly aware of the cost in lost productivity from migraine and other chronic conditions. And though there are no good statistics, there seems to be a growing trend among companies to institute headache clinics. These clinics have a two-pronged focus: educating HR personnel, executives, and employees about the debilitating effects of headaches, particularly the migraine, and educating people who get migraines about treatments.

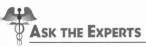

ASK THE EXPERTS

I am between jobs and don't have any health insurance right now. How do I find inexpensive health insurance that will cover my migraine?

You want to consider health insurance coverage that is based on membership instead of employment. Consider joining a trade or professional organization that has its own health insurance. For example, if you are a graphic artist, you can join the AIGA, the American Institute of Graphic Artists. It has an insurance plan for its members, and once you join you can become eligible for coverage.

I have had to miss a couple of days of a workshop due to a migraine. Should I tell my boss about my migraine?

This is totally up to you. It is not necessary to go public about your health to your employer, unless your performance at work is suffering because of it. Only you can know that. Everyone gets sick from time to time. You should not be made to feel guilty about taking your allotted sick days. If you find you need more time off because of your migraine, then yes, you do need to explain your situation to your boss. See pages 188–189 on how to talk about having a chronic illness. You need to work with your boss to accommodate both your health needs and the needs of the business.

Managing the inconveniences
dealing with the hard issues

There are a number of inconveniences involved when you have a chronic illness. They usually come down to two things: time and money. If your symptoms are still troubling you, you are bound to find yourself canceling social engagements or perhaps rearranging your work schedule. Then, of course, there are the many doctor's appointments you need to factor into your already busy schedule. This is not fun.

Next comes a real stressor for those with chronic illnesses: paying for it. If you do not have health insurance, or even if you do have health insurance, having a chronic illness like migraine can result in some out-of-pocket expenses. If you don't respond to low-end analgesics like acetaminophen or ibuprofen, and you don't have prescription coverage, you'll have to pay out-of-pocket for other medications. Migraine-specific medications, like the triptans, are expensive.

Finally, having a chronic illness usually impacts your work life. You may find that you need to cut back on your hours at work from time to time, or find a job that has flexible hours. You should talk to your employer about the nature of your illness, especially if you have severe or frequent migraines.

If you cannot work because of severe, intractable migraines, you can file for disability. If you are fired or if you feel that you are being treated unfairly because you must take some time from work to deal with the migraine, you are protected under the American with Disabilities Act. However, according to the national migraine advocacy group, MAGNUM, "These remedies should be used in only the most serious circumstances, as abuse of such remedies can taint the perception of and the remedies available to other migraine sufferers nationwide."

Learning to live with the migraine

"I spent about five years being stressed about my migraines. My kids felt bad, my husband felt bad, my friends felt bad, and so did I. I was constantly worried about my next episode, so much so that I would cancel outings if I felt even a twinge of pain. Looking back, I lost a lot of time being stressed out—which is kind of funny since I'm a registered nurse and I should know better. The only solution I found was to find a doctor who actually talked to me about my headaches and my worry—in combination. I was not diagnosed with an anxiety disorder or anything, but I was referred to a support group. A lot of the people in the group became my friends. I don't have a magic cure for stress. All I do know is that talking to other people really helped me. Plus, I do go on the Internet and leave messages on migraine boards, especially when I hear about a new treatment or something. I like to listen to other people's opinions, and it's nice to know you're not alone. My only advice is to learn to live with the migraine. I did, and I never thought I'd say that."

—Karen S., Kansas City, KS

Helpful resources

The Chronic Illness Workbook
by Patricia A. Fennel

Who Moved My Cheese? An
Amazing Way to Deal with Change
in Your Work and in Your Life
by Spenser Johnson, M.D., and
Kenneth H. Blanchard

Managing Stress: Principles and
Strategies for Health and Well-Being
(Web Enhanced with CD-ROM)
by Brian Luke Seaward

The Relaxation & Stress Reduction
Workbook
by Martha Davis, et al

Instant Relief: Tell Me Where It
Hurts and I'll Tell You What to Do
by Peggy W. Brill, Susan Suffes

Mind, Stress, and Emotions: The
New Science of Mood
by Gene Wallenstein

www.psychosocialnetwork.org/
faq_stress.htm

www.4woman.gov/faq/

www.yourmedicalsource.com

CHAPTER 12

Living with Migraines

Life with a chronic illness
it can be a rocky road

In your not-too-distant past, whenever you got sick, you went to a doctor, got a prescription, maybe had a little surgery, felt better, and went on with your life. But the migraine—despite modern medicine's best efforts—defies this pattern. Sure, there are treatments that can provide relief. And migraines have been known to stop on their own for women post-menopause. But that's certainly not the case for every female who gets migraines. Men can have migraine episodes well into their senior years. The reality is that for you now, having a chronic illness is normal.

Like other major changes in your life, such as switching careers or becoming a parent, the adjustment to life as a person who gets migraines can be rough. But don't think you're alone. A quick Internet search (see Chapter 7) will show you just how common migraine-inspired frustration can be.

Actually, a diagnosis of a non-terminal illness like the migraine can be a relief. After all, who wouldn't be happy to know they don't have an inoperable brain tumor and are in otherwise good health? But that euphoria can be short-lived and is by no means a universal reaction to the disease called migraine. Many people are overcome with sadness. Others may become angry. And still others resigned. The emotions elicited by chronic illness are similar to the stages of grief. In fact, the newly diagnosed person is grieving over lost health and all the ramifications of that loss.

Living with chronic illness requires an ongoing search for a positive quality of life. For those with a chronic illness there are two goals: dealing with the medical problem itself and coping with the ways that illness affects a life and lifestyle. Those who are most successful in their dealings with a chronic disease eventually find ways to tap their reserves of creativity, intelligence, and perseverance.

Remember, your diagnosis and the changes that come with it throw some big changes at your spouse, too. Your better half can feel a little overwhelmed with all there is to learn. Living with a chronic illness, or with someone who has one, is challenging. And, yes, there will be frustrations. There are several aspects of chronic illness that make it especially difficult for others to understand. One is that migraine isn't visible. It's not like walking around with a broken leg. Or even coping with a life-threatening illness like cancer. People may think, "Get over yourself. It's just a headache." All they will see is you retreating to a darkened bedroom because you can't cope.

There will also be a lack of consistency in your migraines. It's hard for people to truly understand how you can be fine for weeks at a time and then miss days of work or a social activity because you have a headache. You could be as healthy as the proverbial horse in the evening and sick as a dog the next morning. That unpredictability can make both you and your family anxious. All of us are great at rallying around people in an emergency. We're not that good with painful symptoms that strike at will.

Considering all of these factors, it's not surprising that you feel that there's a lack of understanding around you. At the best of times, you need to talk about your feelings, and that's doubly true if you have a chronic illness. You need to learn to talk about the change from the old you to the new you.

The most important thing to remember is that you're not alone. There are some 30 million people who get migraines in the United States; they are young and old, from all walks of life, and the majority are coping with their common illness, leading fulfilling lives. You can, too.

Making the transition
adjusting to a new self-image

A disease like the migraine can affect your life. Even for those with mild to moderate pain, the headaches can require what is seemingly an ongoing quest for the right treatment. And what about those other symptoms like nausea or sensitivity to light? Then there are those changes in lifestyle that you probably will have to make like avoiding certain triggers. And what happens if you don't catch the migraine in time? You probably have to go into a darkened room and lie down and let the migraine take its course. For those individuals who have severe and frequent migraines, there are a host of issues they must contend with. Especially if a treatment plan isn't working. Whatever the case, some times it may be difficult to feel good about yourself when even the slightest movement can make your head pain worse.

Every person who has experienced strange medical symptoms can be very frightened. That's normal. And finding out that you have a chronic condition—even an episodic one like the migraine—can be difficult for some people. For those on a preventive treatment regimen, taking medicine every day is a constant reminder that good health and feeling good every day cannot be taken for granted.

While it may not be clear what lies ahead, there are roadmaps to help you plot the adjustment you need to make. The message is simple: the severity and frequency of migraine varies among individuals, but all those people with migraines are dealing with a chronic condition. There are people who can help. And there are ways that you can help yourself.

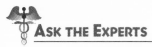

ASK THE EXPERTS

**I overheard my doctor referring to me as a migraineur. I told him I
didn't like to be called that. He was taken aback and said that was
the proper term for a person who gets migraines. Why would such a
little word make me so upset?**

Your doctor is essentially labeling you by your disease, and you rightly
resented that because you are much more than your migraines. It is very
easy to label people by those features that most stand out: their hair
color, their skin color, their job, their sexual preference, even their disease. The problem with any label is that it puts distance between you and
your labeler. Being called by a label makes you feel isolated and alone.
That is probably why you felt so hurt and upset. To be fair, your doctor
is not your friend, per se; she is the medical support person who is
focused exclusively on your migraines. Labels are doubly problematic
if you internalize them. Do not fall for the trap of defining yourself by
your disease.

**I can't decide which is worse, having the pain of a full-blown
migraine or anticipating the pain of one. How do people cope with
the potential pain hanging literally over their heads?**

The threat of pain is a huge stressor. It is so powerful that it can totally
change behavior. Feeling that the onset of pain is beyond your control
can bring on a kind of learned helplessness, leaving you with lower
motivation. But remember that with the right medication and by changing your habits you do have some control over your migraine.

Stages of adjustment
from shock to acceptance

Researchers are discovering that how people cope with the news of chronic illness has a phenomenal effect on long-term physical and emotional health. It's natural to experience what we know as the five stages of grief defined by Dr. Elisabeth Kubler-Ross in her groundbreaking work, *On Death and Dying*. They are denial, anger, bargaining, depression, and acceptance. Take a look at these stages to see where you are. There is no magic bullet to move more quickly from one stage to the next. But there are things you can do to ease each of the transitions.

Denial

Once you get the diagnosis, you realize that migraine is something you always need to be aware of. For some people, especially those with severe and frequent migraines, and even those people who have milder forms of migraine but who have multiple triggers or a treatment plan that isn't working, it can be tough to make lifestyle adjustments, such as taking medication and even avoiding triggers. Not surprisingly, some people often choose to ignore migraine, hoping that it may just go away. What's the reason for this? For most people, it's fear. There is a loss of personal power, of self-esteem. There is also a loss of independence because your migraine inevitably interferes with how you want to manage your life. Going back to your doctor for a new treatment plan seems futile, or so you think. You opt to deny any problems. But if you're not careful, denial can become dangerous defiance. "I'll just take a vacation, or some time off from work!" you might tell yourself, or: "I'll just take more ibuprofen." But remember the rebound! (See page 58.)

What to do?

♦ Think through the situation. What would you tell a friend who was experiencing severe headaches? Probably the same thing your family and friends are telling you. Seek help. Don't self-diagnose.

Anger, Depression, and Bargaining

You're mad at everything and everyone. "I see my doctor for checkups. I give to animal welfare groups. I am a good person. This just isn't fair!" Your friends, family, and colleagues go on as if your migraine isn't any big deal. You know you don't have a serious illness with a capital "S", and you're not going to die from this thing—but you feel depressed since no one seems to understand what you are going through. You may even want to bargain your way out of a migraine. "If I avoid my migraine triggers and take my medication, I'll never have another migraine," is an all-too-common refrain.

What to do?

You will have to remind yourself that you'll have some great days and some not-so-great days, and there is no such thing as total recovery. Migraine is with you daily because there is no cure. One important fact to remember is that contrary to what's commonly believed, the majority of people living with chronic illnesses are not elderly or disabled. More than half are between the ages of 18 and 64, and few report they limit their activities solely based on their disease.

Acceptance

Having gone through some or all of the previous stages, you now accept your illness as part of yourself, a reality to be lived with, not escaped. You recognize that your best chance for future happiness lies in your understanding of the condition and your disciplined commitment to its control.

Beyond acceptance
your job now is to recreate your life

Learning to accept a chronic disorder as part of your life is not easy. You miss the old carefree you. You miss not having to think about your health. You now fully understand why your grandparents used to say, "Don't take your health for granted." And you know what you have to do. With that knowledge comes a certain amount of power. It gives you back control over your life. Yes, you have this disorder, but it is treatable and it need not define who you are. You are still you, just a bit different thanks to your migraine. Yes, it is a different life than the one you had originally planned before you got this problem, but that's okay. The point is to work with this new reality and make it your own. Here are some helpful suggestions.

Learn About Your Condition

Becoming a student of your condition can be an important way to know what is going on with your body. Use as many sources as you can to gather information so you understand what doctors are doing to help you. Learn about your medications and watch for their side effects. Follow doctors' instructions and keep focused on the goal—dealing with the disease. In this information age, it would seem easy to access knowledge, but be cautious. Myths about migraine can spread quickly. Family and friends can be well-intentioned but often offer unsolicited advice. Decide how much contact you want with people, because with so much advice, it can feel as if you're not doing the right thing.

Take Control

The most successful migraine patients are those who are active participants in their treatment. That means you can choose who will treat you, and change your doctor if you feel your migraine is not getting the attention it deserves. You can discuss how often follow-up visits may occur to see if a migraine treatment plan is working. You can ask questions. And get answers. The message is: Be involved.

Find the Right Doctor

In the beginning, it's important to find the right doctor. Don't be afraid to insist on a doctor who understands you and communicates clearly. After all, this is a person who will be helping you regain your life. You need to have a good relationship, so find someone who will collaborate with you and take an interest in you and your care.

Beginning the journey
taking it step by step

After a diagnosis, no one is certain what the final outcome will be. It's hard to live with this new, and constant, level of uncertainty and ambiguity. But how you cope and live with this can make all the difference. What seems undoable and unmanageable is doable. To combat the chaos, new patients can follow a few smart strategies. One is to obtain as much information as possible. Finding out the facts can help relieve anxiety and lessen the fear of the unknown. Besides, knowledge helps the patient regain control and make informed decisions.

Identify and Avoid Vicious Cycles

For example, having high blood pressure from heart disease may make a person feel discouraged, and being discouraged may contribute to feelings of uselessness. These feelings, in turn, can contribute to a sense of fatigue, which then may increase the feeling of being useless and unhappy. This is classic vicious-cycle behavior.

Be Positive

Trying to figure out new ways to enjoy old activities is fine, but if you are feeling depressed, it also helps to focus on things that you can still do well. Remember that you are a competent, unique person—with many talents and attributes that are still yours.

- Use laughter and humor to reduce stress.

- Build on the talents and activities you can still enjoy.

- Pay attention to your body. How does it feel? How is it reacting to the things you are doing right now? Plan your day accordingly.

- Learn more about yourself. What makes you tense? What makes you want to throw caution to the wind and eat a box of chocolates or slurp three glasses of wine?

Educate

Teach your family, friends, and co-workers about migraine. Many companies have on-site headache seminars. Perhaps you can start one at your work. Talk to your family about what you need, what you expect from treatment, and what to do if those meds don't work on occasion.

◆ Stick to your goals. Migraine is just a migraine, a neurovascular event. Your goals should not diminish because you have migraines. Work toward living your life as if a migraine really is nothing more than a bad headache.

Get Help

Find other people who get migraines if that kind of support is what you need. Though friends, co-workers, and family can be sympathetic, no one knows the pain of the migraine better than those who experience these episodic hellraisers. There are many support groups online, and there may be some "live" support groups in your area. Check out local hospitals to see if they offer migraine support.

Dealing with setbacks
bumps along the way

Migraines can feel like a never-ending series of speed bumps. Between the surreal pre-migraine feelings to the throbbing headache to the recovery phase, you can feel as if you are on a roller coaster. And then just when you've been dealing with all your new physical and mental changes, wham, your migraines start getting worse or more frequent, or some other troubling health condition pops up. It's as if you are starting all over again from scratch.

This is part and parcel of having a chronic illness. Try to remember that having a chronic illness calls for a different way of looking at your health. It is no longer this static thing you can rely upon. You will have good days as well as bad days. And sometimes those bad days can be horrendous. This unpredictability is to be expected. If it's any comfort, you are not alone. Over half of the population of America, that's almost 150 million people, have some kind of chronic health problem. And 30 million of them have migraine.

What do you do? How do you cope? For starters, call the members of your support team and check out your current situation with them. Then go to your safe haven (see page 180) and regroup. You may need to cut back on your activities and social life for a bit. But you will be back in form soon. Load up on good books and funny movies. A hearty laugh can help get you over tough spots. Connect with family and friends and let them know what you need. Don't expect them to be able to read your mind and know that you want some TLC or need downtime. Tell them.

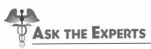

ASK THE EXPERTS

How do I handle important meetings and social events when I feel a migraine coming on?

There are a number of prescription medications on the market that are designed to interrupt a migraine before it becomes a full-blown assault. The triptans (see pages 52-53) seem to be especially helpful with this. Some people carry an emergency triptan injection or pill just for these occasions. Failing that, all you can do is have a backup plan in case you cannot make it.

Becoming an Advocate

Giving back by helping others
One of the many things having a chronic illness can do is to teach you how to accept help with grace. For many people this is the hardest lesson. Our culture thrives on independence. Those who ask for help are often chided for being lazy or inept. Another reason it's hard to ask for help is that many of us have internalized those voices of derision that say we are bad for asking. And so we don't ask, or if we do, we feel ashamed about it.

Having a chronic illness changes all that. You have no choice but to ask for help. And over time, you learn that there is nothing kinder and more loving than help kindly given. Small wonder that people who have undergone great physical and emotional trials are the ones who give back to others who are suffering.

There are many ways you can give back. You can go online and add your knowledge to the various support groups on the Internet that provide so much help to those in the throes of early diagnosis (see page 120 for Web addresses). You can also join the various nonprofit organizations that support migraine research. You can volunteer to help with their newsletters and other activities. Becoming an advocate is a great way to share your illness story with others.

Helpful resources

The Chronic Illness Workbook
by Pat Fennell

On Death and Dying
by Elisabeth Kubler-Ross

Recrafting a Life
by Charlie Johnson and
Denise Webster

On Being Ill
by Virginia Woolf

Illness as Metaphor
by Susan Sontag

Glossary

Words in bold type are defined elsewhere in the glossary.

Acupuncture A therapy used in Traditional Chinese Medicine in which fine needles are inserted into specific places in the body to relieve pain and promote healing.

Adrenaline *See:* epinephrine.

Amines Organic substances derived from ammonia. They are found in food or made in the body and help to regulate mood and the diameter of the blood vessels, among other functions. *See also:* epinephrine, histamine, norepinephrine, serotonin, tyramine.

Analgesic Drugs—especially nonprescription drugs such as aspirin, acetaminophen, ibuprofen, or naproxen sodium—that are used to relieve pain.

Aneurysm An abnormal, localized widening of a blood vessel. Aneurysms are more common in arteries than in veins.

Angiogram, angiography A specialized diagnostic technique in which a radio-opaque substance that X-rays cannot pass through is injected into a vein or artery vessel, and a rapid series of X-rays is taken that reveals the size and shape of the vessel. A cerebral angiogram examines vessels in the brain; a cardiac angiogram examines vessels in the heart.

Antidepressant A therapy or medication that prevents, eases, or cures persistent, pervasive sadness. Antidepressant medications, usually available only by prescription, are useful in treating migraine because they help to regulate **amine** levels, which influences the diameter of blood vessels.

Antiemetic drugs Medications that relieve or prevent nausea and/or vomiting.

Aura Symptoms especially visual disturbances, that precede the headache phase in classic migraine. In some people who get migraines, aura does not progress to a painful headache, and these symptoms comprise the episode.

Beta-blockers Formally known as beta-adrenergic blockers, this class of drugs is typically used by people with heart disease. The medication helps keep blood vessels from dilating and, if taken daily, also helps to reduce the incidence or severity of migraine.

Beta-adrenergic blockers *See:* Beta-blockers.

Biofeedback A stress-reduction technique in which people learn how to influence or control some usually involuntary physical processes such as heart rate, blood pressure, and skin temperature. Electronic sensors and a monitor provide the "feedback," and a technician acts as a coach to help you learn to regulate your body's response to tension-producing stimuli.

Calcium-channel blockers Calcium is one of the biological minerals that muscles, including the muscles in the walls of your arteries, use when they contract. Calcium-channel blockers are medications that keep excess calcium from entering the muscle and help to prevent the spasms and vasoconstriction that can trigger migraine. They are most effective when taken daily as a prophylactic, or preventive, treatment and are also used to treat high blood pressure and heart disease.

CAT scan Short for "computerized axial tomography," a CAT scan is a diagnostic test that uses a series of X-ray beams to examine thin cross-sections of the brain. In migraine, a CAT scan will usually show no abnormalities such as bleeding or tumors. A CAT scan is sometimes called a CT scan (the acronym of "computerized tomography").

Cephalalgia, cephalgia Headache or head pain (kephale, Greek for "head" + alosa, "pain").

Classic migraine A category of migraine in which the headache phase is preceded or accompanied by visual disturbances (aura), speech disturbances, dizziness, tingling, numbness, confusion, nausea, or mood changes. These premonitory symptoms are called a prodrome. Classic migraine is also called migraine with aura.

Cluster headache A kind of recurrent headache in which the pain, often intense, is localized around one eye or temple and appears in bouts (clusters) that may persist for 15 minutes or for up to three hours. The bouts are also cyclic and may occur every other day or several times a day for weeks or months, then go into remission, possibly for years, before recurring. Cluster headache is also called migrainous neuralgia or Horner's syndrome.

Common migraine A category of migraine in which the headache arises without a prodrome (warning symptoms such as the visual disturbances that characterize classic migraine). Common migraine is also called migraine without aura.

Computerized Transverse Axial Tomography *See*: CAT scan.

CT scan *See*: CAT scan.

Diuretic Commonly called water pills, diuretics are medications that reduce body fluid by encouraging urination.

Edema Swelling that occurs when the body retains excessive fluid in its tissues.

EEG Short for "electroencephalo-gram," an EEG is a recording the brain's electrical activity. The recording is made by sensors attached to the scalp.

Electroencephalography *See:* EEG.

Electroencephalogram *See:* EEG.

Endorphins A group of powerful analgesic biochemicals with mor-phine-like properties that are pro-duced naturally in the brain.

Epinephrine Sometimes called adrenaline, epinephrine is an amine produced by the adrenal glands. It relaxes the bronchioles (air ducts) to increase respiration, constricts blood vessels to regulate blood pres-sure and the pulse rate, and sup-ports carbohydrate metabolism. Epinephrine also plays a role in the "fight or flight" response; excess lev-els in the blood are implicated in some anxiety disorders.

Ergotamine, ergotamine tartrate A medication made from ergot, a fungus that grows on rye, that con-stricts blood vessels and is useful in treating migraine.

Estrogen A female sex hormone. Decreasing levels just before men-struation can trigger migraine in some women.

Hemicrania Literally "half the head" (hemi, "half" + kranion,

"skull"), the word describes pain on one side of the head, usually migraine pain.

Hemiplegia, hemiplegic migraine Paralysis or weakness on one side of the body. This is a rare symptom of migraine and usually occurs in peo-ple whose tendency to have migraine is inherited. The paralysis is temporary and leaves when the headache resolves. But if you experi-ence this symptom, go to an emer-gency room right away; it could be a stroke.

Histamine An amine normally present in the body that, when acti-vated, causes capillaries and other blood vessels to dilate and produces localized edema.

Hypoglycemia Lower-than-normal amount of sugar in the blood. It may be a trigger for migraine and can cause sweating, light-headed-ness, difficulty concentrating, and headache (other than migraine).

Lumbar puncture The formal term for a spinal tap, lumbar puncture is a diagnostic test done with a local anesthetic. The puncture is made by inserting a fine needle through the lower back into the bottom of the spinal cord. The needle may be used either to extract (tap) spinal fluid for analysis or to inject a contrast medium for particular diagnostic X rays. If fluid is tapped, it is exam-ined for signs of cancer, infection, or bleeding.

Magnetic resonance imaging *See:* MRI.

MAOIs *See*: Monoamine oxidase inhibitors.

Migraine A headache with severe throbbing pain that typically afflicts one side of the head (hemicrania). The headache may persist for up to 72 hours and may or may not be accompanied by symptoms such as visual disturbances (blurred vision, seeing sparks or zigzags of light); hypersensitivity to light, sound, smell, and touch; numbness or tingling; pallor; sweating; and nausea and/or vomiting. The headache is thought to be caused by dilation of the cranial arteries. Susceptibility to migraine tends to run in families. *See also:* Classic migraine, Common migraine, Photophobia.

Migraine with aura *See*: Classic migraine.

Migraine without aura *See*: Common migraine

Migraineur, migraineuse The formal term for a man (migraineur) or a woman (migraineuse) who suffers from migraine.

Migrainous neuralgia *See*: Cluster headache.

Monoamine oxidase inhibitors Abbreviated as MAOIs or MAO inhibitors, this is a class of medicine used to treat depression as well as to prevent migraine. Monoamine oxidase is an enzyme that breaks down monoamines such as **serotonin**, **epinephrine**, and **norepinephrine**.

MRI The acronym for "magnetic resonance imaging," an MRI is a diagnostic test that provides images of soft tissue by inducing the protons and neutrons in the nuclei of atoms in the body to react (resonate) with a strong external magnetic field. The magnetic field is created with radiofrequency pulses, and the images are a result of the degree to which the protons and neutrons absorb or deflect the magnetization. An MRI offers more detail than a **CAT scan**, and as with that test, in migraine the results are usually negative.

Neuralgia Pain arising from an irritated, inflamed, compressed, or injured nerve. Nerve pain is burning, severe, and unrelenting. **Vascular** pain (pain from throbbing blood vessels) is more common in migraine.

Neurogenic Originating in the nervous system or arising from nervous impulses. (For example, fever usually results from infection, but you may have a fever during a migraine as a result of nervous excitation.)

Neurotransmitter A biochemical, such as **norepinephrine**, that passes between two nerve endings and carries (transmits) information that allows or prevents the initiation of electrical impulses in the second cell.

Nonsteroidal anti-inflammatory drugs Abbreviated as NSAIDs, these medications have **analgesic,** anti-inflammatory, and antipyretic (fever-reducing) properties. Many NSAIDs, such as aspirin, acetaminophen, and ibuprofen, are available without a prescription.

Noradrenaline *See*: Norepinephrine.

Norepinephrine A hormone produced by the adrenal glands. It is a **vasoconstrictor** and its effects are similar to those of **epinephrine** but less marked. Norepinephrine is also known as noradrenaline.

NSAIDs *See*: Nonsteroidal anti-inflammatory drugs.

Ophthalmoplegia migraine, ophthalmic migraine A migraine headache with symptoms that include partial or complete paralysis of eye movement or double vision. (The paralysis is a rare and transient symptom and is due to a disorder of the eyes' controls in the brain.)

PET scan Short for "positron emission tomography," this is a test that measures the rate of metabolism by marking a substance such as glucose with an isotope that emits positrons (particles that have the same mass as a negative electron but a positive

charge). Cross-sectional images are taken to track the rate at which the marked substance is disseminated through and used up in the brain.

Photophobia Heightened sensitivity or aversion to light.

Positron emission tomography *See*: PET scan.

Prodrome Symptoms that precede a migraine headache; often these include nausea, vision changes, numbness or tingling, trembling or weakness, and throbbing temples.

Progesterone A female sex hormone. Levels of the hormone decrease before the onset of menstruation and increase during the second half of the menstrual cycle and during pregnancy. Hormonal fluctuations may trigger migraine in some women. *See also*: Estrogen.

Prophylactic medication A medication taken daily to prevent migraine headaches from occurring. *See also*: Beta blockers, Calcium channel blockers.

Prostaglandins A group of biologically active fatty acids with functions similar to those of hormones. Among other things, prostaglandins influence fluid balance, blood flow, neurotransmission, and gastrointestinal function and activity. Because they also have an effect on the caliber of the blood vessels, they are implicated in migraine.

Scotoma (plural: **scotomata**)
Disturbances in vision or the visual
field. In migraine, scotomata are the
most common symptom after
headache, the most common form is
scintillating or flittering scotoma—
shimmering, twinkling, luminous
spots that float across the field of
vision. A scotoma may also appear
as a blank area, gap, or dark spot in
the visual field.

Serotonin A **neurotransmitter**
and potent **vasoconstrictor**, serotonin is found in the brain, blood,
and gastrointestinal mucosa. It is
implicated in migraine and in affec-
tive disorders such as depression.
Serotonin levels increase prior to a
migraine attack and decrease once
the headache begins.

Sinus headache, sinusitis When
the sinuses cannot drain properly
because of inflammation (as from
an allergy) or an infection, a painful
migraine-like headache may occur
(along with fever, nasal congestion,
runny nose, and colored discharge)

Temporal arteritis Chronic
inflammation of the large arteries in
the scalp, especially the temporal
arteries at the sides of the head, the
occipital arteries at the base of the
skull, or the ophthalmic arteries
that serve the eyes. It occurs in people over 50 and, if left untreated,
can lead to blindness.

**Temporomandibular joint syn-
drome** *See*: TMJ syndrome.

Tension headache Head pain that
arises from muscle spasm or from
chronic muscle contraction. Tension
headaches are distinct from
migraine in that the pain is felt on
both sides of the head, it does not
worsen with physical movement,
and sufferers are not nauseated. The
headache may recur in episodes
lasting from minutes to days and
may be more severe, frequent, or
long-lived if the sufferer is under
stress.

Thermography A diagnostic test
that monitors blood flow by measuring the amount of heat present in
the area being studied. (Heat is a
byproduct of chemical reactions in
the body.)

TMJ syndrome Severe migrainous
pain that comes from clenching the
jaw or grinding the teeth. The jaw
hinge, the temporomandibular joint,
becomes stiff and painful and may
make clicking sounds (especially
during chewing). Tinnitus or deaf-
ness may also be present. ("TMJ" is
an abbreviation for "temporomandibular joint.")

Trigeminal neuralgia Pain that
arises from the trigeminal nerve, the
nerve that supplies sensation to the
face; may be confused with
migraine or other headache pain.

Trigger An item or event that leads to a migraine headache. Triggers are individual to the people who experience them and include dietary, environmental, chemical, or hormonal substances, as well as emotional factors such as stress (or the letdown period from stress) and changes in one's usual routine.

Tyramine An **amine** found in aged cheese and other foods that produces **vasodilation** and migraine in susceptible individuals.

Vascular Pertaining to the blood vessels.

Vasoconstriction, vasoconstrictor A narrowing of the blood vessels; a substance, such as **serotonin** or **ergotamine**, that causes blood vessels to constrict.

Vasodilation, vasodilator A widening of the blood vessels; a substance, such as **histamine**, that causes blood vessels to dilate. (Vasodilation is sometimes given as "vasodilatation.")

Vertigo The sensation of movement when there is none, thus a hallucination of movement.

Index